all you need to kn(
HAIR, SKIN AND BEA

(THE COMPLETE BOL

all you need to know about HAIR, SKIN & BEAUTY CARE
(THE COMPLETE BODY BOOK)

Blossom Kochhar

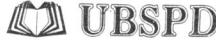
UBS Publishers' Distributors Ltd.
New Delhi • Bombay • Bangalore • Madras
Calcutta • Patna • Kanpur • London

UBS Publishers' Distributors Ltd.
5 Ansari Road, New Delhi-110 002
Bombay Bangalore Madras Calcutta Patna Kanpur London

© Blossom Kochhar

First Published	1992
First Reprint	1993
Second Reprint	1993
Third Reprint	1993
Fourth Reprint	1993
Fifth Reprint	1993
Sixth Reprint	1994
Seventh Reprint	1995
Eighth Reprint	1996

All rights reserved. No part of this publication may be reproduced or transmitted in any form or by any means, electronic or mechanical, including photocopying, recording or any information storage or retrieval system, without prior permission in writing from the publisher.

Cover Design : UBS Art Studio.

Lasertypeset at Rajkamal Electric Press
Printed at Nutech Photolithographers
Shahdara Delhi-110 095

*To my mother and father
Albert and Marie Otter
&
Leo Passage*

Contents

Preface	ix

The Hair Section

1.	Understanding hair and its care	1
2.	Conditioning your hair	12
3.	Dandruff	17
4.	Dealing with falling hair	21
5.	Colouring your hair	28
6.	Selecting hair style	34
7.	Caring for long hair	41
8.	Perming hair	44
9.	Managing your hair	47

The Skin Section

10.	Understanding the skin and its care	51
11.	Improving the skin complexion and texture	76
12.	Dealing with acne	83
13.	Closing the open pores	96
14.	Clearing up pigmentation	100
15.	Seasonal skin care	107
16.	Make-up	117

The Body Section

17.	The all of you	125

18.	Treating cellulite	135
19.	Hands	141
20.	Your pedestals—the feet	146
21.	Ridding yourself of superfluous hair	151
22.	Nutrition and diet	156
23.	Figuring out the diet	159
24.	Exercises	168

Appendix I   173

Appendix II   176

Preface

Over the years I have researched and written something in the region of one to two thousand articles, features, and booklets on every aspect of beauty. I have written about skin and hair, figure, food, diets and nutrition, on exercising, ageing and staying young and healthy, and on beauty problems of every conceivable kind.

Lecturing to groups of women, and answering personal questions afterwards, as well as dealing with thousands of letters from readers has convinced me that every girl and every woman has beauty problems of some kind, no matter how poised and sophisticated she may appear to the world at large.

Income, position, status, education and age have little or nothing to do with the matter. School girls may worry about spots, mature women will want to delay the onset of lines but there are countless other women with innumerable anxieties.

This book is an attempt to answer beauty problems as they arise and where possible to prevent others occurring.

Because I have literally spent the past 20 years, eight hours a day, in a salon, I've got notebooks filled with the "How to" perfected techniques that will explain, step by step, how you can make them work for you at home.

The book is divided into three comprehensive parts *Hair, Skin* and *Body* which provide in-depth answers to many of the behind-closed-doors questions you've never been able to bring yourself to ask.

I was determined to present new facts about the nitty-gritties, because if I've learnt one thing from my frequent talks/demonstrations it's this: Today, women no longer believe that beauty can be bought in a jar (I don't believe it, and cosmetics are my business, so why should you?). Women want the whole picture, and they're not embarrassed to ask me questions about the nitty-gritties, such as:

- How to get rid of acne scars.
- How to lose weight without going crazy.
- How to remove unwanted hair—professionally.
- How to get rid of those spidery lines on legs.
- The good news and the bad news about skin and hair care, colouring, diet, exercise, and more.

The girls and women I've spoken to want sensible advice. That's what this book provides.

I would like to thank Sanjiv Channan for helping me with this book. Also my husband and daughter, and my colleagues at Pivot Point.

New Delhi   BLOSSOM KOCHHAR

Three Golden Principles of Beauty Care

- Use as little cosmetics as possible. Keep your skin and hair naturally beautiful.
- Avoid using chemically-prepared and preserved cosmetics.
- Use natural cosmetics personally made at home from herbs, fruits and vegetables. Try and make them fresh before use.

THE HAIR SECTION

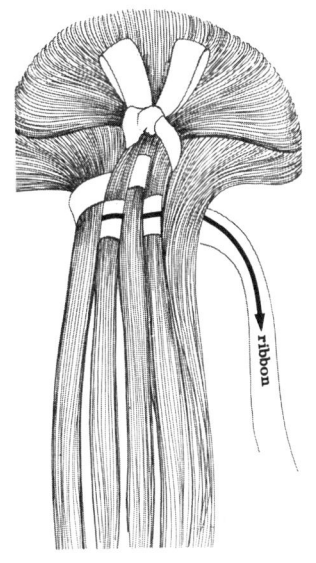

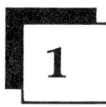

Understanding Hair and its Care

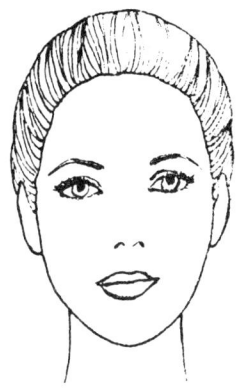

Hair is the most versatile and a permanent accessory of a woman. It is a vital part of her looks and her personality. Hair gives a frame to a woman's face, complements her lifestyle, accentuates her fashion appeal and more. To a cosmopolitan woman, hair is a fluid medium of self-expression and art.

Any woman who appreciates good looks and great hairstyles also recognises the merit in taking good care of it. It surely makes taking good care of hair a lot easier and resultful if one *understands* hair—its structure, its characteristics, the condition of the scalp it grows on, etc.

THE STRUCTURE OF HAIR AND ITS GROWTH

Hair is made of strong elastic strands of protein called *keratin* and in chemical terms is composed of oxygen, iron, nitrogen, hydrogen, sulphur, carbon and phosphorus. The exact proportions of these chemical elements vary with sex, age, type and colour of hair.

The sources of hair are very small tiny pockets in our skin and scalp known as *follicles*. These follicles are not evenly spread on the scalp but are found together in groups of two to five each. Every follicle follows a life cycle of its own, producing six inches of hair a year, for as long as four years, before it falls out, then starts all over again after a short period.

The basal tip of the hair in the scalp is known as *papilla*, which is a small out-growth of the skin, shaped like a doorknob and lying at the tip of the follicle. The papilla contains the blood vessels to supply nourishment to the hair.

During the active period, the new cell growth pushes the older part of the hair away from the papilla until the hair falls out. It is the pattern of cell growth at the papilla which determines whether hair grow straight, wavy or curly.

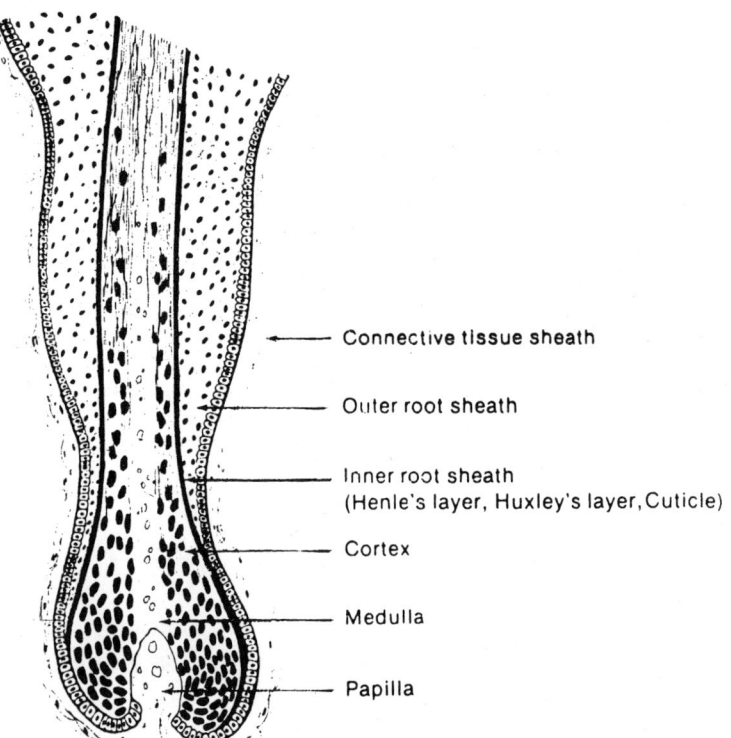

The growth pattern usually becomes uneven during the adolescence when the hair growth is at its peak. It declines as we grow older. The cell growth pattern can change otherwise also due to illness, drugs, pregnancy, etc.

Though hair strands look as singular fibres, each hair is constructed in three different layers: the *cuticle*, the *cortex* and the *medulla*.

The cuticle is the outermost layer of the hair which provides protection to the inner cortex layer. It is made up of flattened, hard, horny cells. When the cuticle breaks and dislodges at the end of the hair, the result is split ends. Improper care and frequent use of harsh chemicals on hair damage the cuticle.

The cortex is the second layer. The qualitative properties of strength, elasticity, pliability, direction and growth pattern, width and the texture of hair depend on the composition of the cortex. The cortex is composed of fibres twisted together like a rope.

It is the cortex which gives the hair its colour. The presence of the four natural pigments black, brown, yellow and red are logged in the cortex in varying proportions, and the air spaces in the cortex determine the colour and shade of hair. The excess black and deep brown pigment is what gives oriental women the dark hair they possess.

Lastly, the medulla is the unimportant innermost layer which is composed of soft keratin. Medulla is often not present in some hair. Hair that lacks medulla is no worse than hair that has medulla.

THE CHARACTERISTICS OF HEALTHY HAIR

It may surprise you, but till date, no cosmetologist or trichologist has been able to comprehensively and conclusively describe all the characteristics of healthy hair. Some of the most common characteristics of healthy hair quoted are:

- Thick and dense.
- Fine and silky, which means not too oily or rough.
- Lustre-filled, having a shine and gloss.
- Pliable, capable of setting and styling.
- Full-bodied and not limp or lank.

While describing the condition of hair, it is important to keep in mind, the hair growth. Unless the growth is proper and regular, the hair condition is considered affected.

REGULAR CARE OF HAIR

Taking care of hair is in fact much the same as taking care of skin. An effective hair-care discipline involves cleansing, toning and conditioning routines carried out with religious regularity.

Another important aspect of effective care is the use of proper hair-care products. Different types of hair need different hair-care products. The use of wrong products is detrimental to the hair.

Cleansing is the foremost routine in daily hair care. The purpose of cleansing is to wash away excess oil on hair and scalp and clear the hair follicles off the debris of unexfoliated dead cells. Proper cleansing encourages healthy hair growth.

After cleansing, the scalp and hair need the toning exercise. The toning of scalp and hair is achieved by gently massaging the head. This helps in stimulating and invigorating the blood circulation required for the healthy growth of hair.

The most important part of hair-care is conditioning. It is a restorative routine. If the hair is excessively stripped of moisture or oil due to harsh cleansing, sun or application of harsh chemicals such as perm lotions, etc., the conditioning routine aims at restoring and correcting the imbalance. The kind of conditioning required depends entirely on the physical condition of the hair.

FACTORS AFFECTING HAIR

The condition of hair is directly linked to the physiological well-being of our bodies. Apart from improper hair-care, there are several other factors that can be detrimental to hair.

Here is a list of those factors:

- Hereditary/genes also determine the hair colour and density.
- Chemical and drug reactions.
- Hormonal changes.
- Emotional stress, trauma.

These factors, by and large, influence the hair condition and its proper growth. We will examine them when we discuss the hair disorders in succeeding chapters.

TYPES OF HAIR AND SCALP CONDITIONS

There are basically three types of hair: oily, dry and normal.

Oily Hair

When the oil glands (Sebaceous glands) in the scalp secrete excess oil, it travels down the hair shaft, causing excessive oiliness on the scalp and hair. The oily hair appears lank, dark and coarse.

Dry Hair

In contrast to the oily hair condition, dry hair is a result of the lack of sebum and oil on the hair causing it to dry out at cellular level. Flakiness of the scalp and dandruff are a direct result of dryness. The hair looks limp, becomes less elastic and is more susceptible to breakage and damage.

Normal Hair

It is healthy, silky hair without over-dry ends or over-oily roots. It is the easiest to cope and care for.

CARE OF OILY HAIR AND SCALP CONDITION

The principle of care for oily hair and scalp condition is the same as used for oily skin condition.

The hair routine aims at removing the excess oil and to exfoliate skin cells which clog up and suffocate the hair follicles in our scalp. Infection usually erupts in the blocked hair follicles which leads to hair loss and other scalp disorders.

The emphasis is laid on cleansing and toning routines. The cleansing routine involves washing and rinsing the hair. Since the hair has to be washed as frequently as it gets dirty and oily, a natural shampoo on a formulation of herbs such as *amla, shikakai, trifla* is ideal.

The ideal shampoo is always gentle in action, thorough in dissolving the grime and at the same time, not harsh like a detergent shampoo.

Massaging hair and scalp is important for the well-being as well as good growth of the hair. For dry hair, scalp massaging with oil is recommended. For oily hair, massage with toning lotion is suitable. A two minute brushing, stroking and combing routine is sufficient massage exercise for the scalp.

THE HOME-MADE COSMETIC CARE FOR OILY HAIR

There are some very simple and effective recipes that work wonderfully if followed as advised.

Shampoo Cleanser Recipe

- Buy some *shikakai* powder from the market. Powder some *green grams* and *fenugreek* (*methi*) seeds. Mix two portions of *shikakai* powder, one portion of green gram flour and half portion of Fenugreek powder and keep it. When required, mix a tablespoon of this mixture in the white of an egg and use it as a shampoo. It does not lather like a soap, or shampoo, but cleanses the hair.
- Take some dry soap nuts (*reetha*) and soak them in water overnight. Mash them in the morning and strain the soapy solution. Add a teaspoon of *shikakai* powder and wash your hair.

A Mint Infusion Recipe

- If you are unable to make the shampoo cleanser at home, use this infusion recipe. Prepare it and mix it in the shampoo you use.

To make the infusion, boil two handfuls of mint (*pudina*) in one-and-a-half glass of water for 20 minutes. Strain the solution and mix in a 300 ml bottle of shampoo.

The Toning Lotion

- Mix a tablespoon of Malt Vinegar in a glass of water. Add a pinch of salt in it. Dab two tablespoons of it on your scalp and massage it with your finger tips twice a week. Leave the lotion on for one hour. Rinse with cool water, brush and set your hair.

Other Tips

- Do not use detergent shampoos.
- Do not use oils unless the cleansing routine leaves your hair extremely dry.
- Regularly massage your scalp.

CARE OF DRY HAIR

Dry hair tends to be thin and rough. It is susceptible to tangles, damage, breakage and split ends.

The primary aim is to replenish the oil and the moisture in the hair. That is why the emphasis is on the conditioning aspect of hair care. Strong cleansing routines and dry toning exercises and massaging of the scalp promote dryness and flakiness of the scalp.

The use of strong-action shampoo is prohibited for dry hair. Often a generous oil application and massage is recommended before washing the hair. Frequent shampooing is harmful for dry hair.

For the moisture-dry hair, a moisturiser application is required.

THE HOME-MADE COSMETIC CARE FOR DRY HAIR

Below are given few natural recipes that are time-tested. For maximum result, use these recipes regularly in place of chemical products.

The Gentle Cleanser

- Beat an egg in a cup of skimmed milk. When the foam becomes consistent, rub it into the scalp. Leave it on for 5 minutes. Rinse the hair thoroughly with water. Carry out this routine twice a week.
- Take a cup of coconut milk and add two tablespoons of gram flour or one teaspoon of *shikakai*. Apply on your scalp and hair and massage gently. Rinse it out after five minutes. Follow this recipe atleast once a week.

The Protein Conditioner

Beat one tablespoon of castor oil, one tablespoon of glycerine, a teaspoon of cider vinegar and a teaspoon of protein, plus a tablespoon of mild herbal shampoo. Apply it on scalp and leave it on for 20 minutes. Rinse with clear water.

A Special Massage Oil/Toner

Buy a bottle of castor oil or coconut oil. Add a teaspoon of lavender essential oil in it. Heat a little and massage it gently in your scalp at night. Rinse or shampoo it out in the morning. Follow this routine atleast twice a week.

In my years of experience, I have found all the above recipes potent and helpful.

Other Tips

- First assess whether your scalp and hair are moisture-dry or oil-dry.
- Condition your hair as often as you wash it.
- Never comb, brush or massage vigorously if the hair is extremely dry.

Before any kind of routine care is followed, I reiterate, be familiar with the needs of *your* scalp and hair.

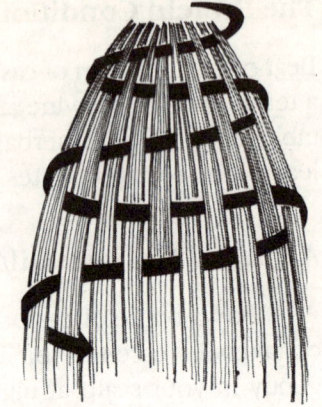

2

Conditioning Your Hair

Our hair suffers from the abuses rendered by the city environment—the air is polluted, the water we drink and wash our hair with is laden with chemicals. That's not all, the suffering is worsened by the harsh and strong hair-care with chemical cosmetics, emotional crisis, hormonal problems and adverse weather conditions. All these cause the problems of split ends, dryness or oiliness, limpness, or frizzy unmanageability. This is when a conditioner comes to your rescue.

A *conditioner* is a beauty preparation that improves the texture of the hair and makes them easily manageable. It comes in as many different kinds as there are hair problems and is applied mostly after shampoo.

WHY WE SHOULD CONDITION OUR HAIR

Conditioning is a very important aspect of the hair-care routine, almost all kinds of hair need conditioning to some extent or the other. It is carried out to rejuvenate our hair which is usually robbed of its vitality by the abuse it is exposed to.

Conditioning is in fact a restorative routine, and falls in the category of preventive hair-care as explained.

Conditioning Restores Body and Bounce to Limp Hair

There are two kinds of body-building conditioners—the ones you rinse out and the ones you leave in. Both work at adding bulk to the hair by leaving some material on the hair shaft. These materials include polymer fibers and protein.

Conditioning Restores the Acid Mantle and Removes Snarls from the Hair

The special cream rinse conditioners are designed to untangle the frizz in the hair. Many also add the welcome beauty benefit of high gloss to the locks. The cream rinse coats the hair to help minimise the stress on the hair from brushing, combing, setting and keeps breakage and split ends under control. Cream rinses do not add body but only soften the hair.

Conditioning Restores the Damaged Hair into Full-bodied Hair

We use *Deep Conditioners* to help restore the dry, damaged hair, plus hair that is brittle excessively and broken in anyway. The deep conditioners contain large amounts of protein. In order that these proteins are absorbed, the deep conditioner should be applied for a longer time. The protein works by repairing hair damage at the area that is badly in need of help.

Conditioning Helps Restore the Loss of Moisture in Hair

Conditioners also help in reducing friction and adding combability to hair. In addition, they help in removing dryness and moisturising it.

Home-made Cosmetic Care

There are several effective and simple-to-make conditioner recipes. The recipes made at home are not as harsh as the chemical conditioners, and are pure and resultful.

The All-purpose Conditioner Rinse

Mix the following to prepare the magic rinse:

- 1 Teaspoon of castor oil.
- 1 Teaspoon of *Amla* or *Brahmi* oil.
- 1 Teaspoon of *Malt Vinegar*.
- 1 Teaspoon of *Glycerine*.
- 1 Teaspoon of Shampoo.

The castor oil gives body to hair; the herbal oil acts like a hair tonic, vinegar restores the acid mantle, glycerine moisturises the hair and shampoo is the medium that blends the ingredients. Before washing the hair, apply this mixture to the hair gently and leave it on for about twenty minutes. Shampoo it out with clear water and feel the marvellous change in your hair texture.

Conditioner for Shine and Sheen

Grate few onions and some cabbage together and leave in a copper utensil overnight. In the morning, add few drops of eau-de cologne to remove the onion smell. Add few drops of a herbal oil like *Amla* or *Brahmi* and then apply. Shampoo after 20 minutes. Your hair will gain a superb gloss and colour. You may follow this routine once a week.

Henna Conditioners

(a) For oily hair—Mix *Henna* with 2 tablespoons of yogurt and a pinch of sugar to a light paste. Add a bit of water if the paste is thick. Apply on hair and leave it on for twenty minutes. Rinse it out with clear water.

(b) For dry hair—Mix *Henna* in a tablespoon of oil and enough warm milk to make a paste. Apply and leave on for twenty minutes. Rinse it out later.

The *Henna* conditioners give colour sheen and body to the hair.

A Hair–Setting Conditioner

Mix one teaspoon of gelatin, available in the market, in a mug of water. Rinse your hair with it. Finger-dry your hair and set them as you desire.

Because there are different kinds of conditioners, you can be very specific in your choice and use the one that best suits your needs. Use herbal or home-made conditioners preferably.

The Conditioning Prescription at Glance

Hair Condition	Cause	Treatment
Frizzy, out of control	Humidity	Use moisturising cream conditioner.
Limp, flat, brassy	Sweat	Perspiration, a weak acid, takes the life out of hair. Wash it out as soon as you can, with a mild shampoo. For treated hair which turns brassy, try a colour rinse. Add a teaspoon of instant coffee to your conditioner before use.
Faded, dry	Overexposure to sun	Sun strips hair of moisture. Wear a hat; use a hair sunscreen.
Greenish, brittle	Chlorinated pools	Hair absorbs chlorine, metals, which can change hair colour. Combat by using a soda-water rinse. Ease dryness with an oil massage once a week. Use bathing cap.

(Contd.)

16 Hair, Skin and Beauty Care

Hair Condition	Cause	Treatment
Dull, limp unmanageable	Pollution	Dirt from heavy, polluted air clings to hair. Our pollution solution: 1 quart water, 6 oz rose water, 4 oz vinegar. Apply, rinse out, after shampoo twice a month. Use less of everything on your hair.

3

Dandruff

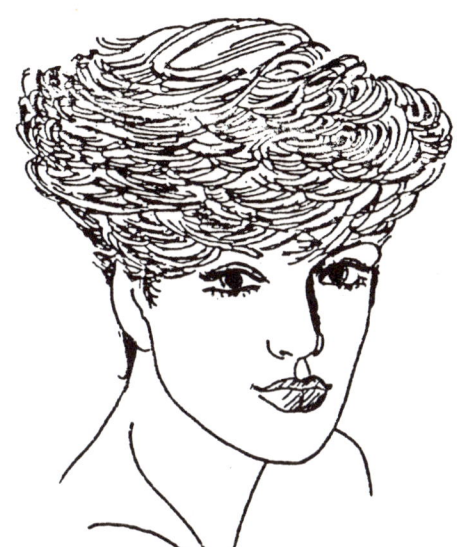

Dandruff is the single most common problem that can occur on every body. To have a few white-flaked cells is normal for it is simply the sloughing off matured skin cells and waste material through the pores of the scalp. It is only when this becomes excessive that it has to be considered a problem. Well-looked after, clean, healthy hair with the proper acid balance does not have problem dandruff.

There are two forms of dandruff—oily and dry. The dry dandruff appears as loose white flakes, and the scalp itches a great deal. The oily dandruff is sticky and yellow in colour, and the scalp with oily dandruff smells bad. The oily form is found most among adolescents and adults with an excessively oily skin and scalp.

WHAT CAUSES DANDRUFF

The basic causes of dandruff are faulty diet, emotional tension and stress, hormonal disturbances, infection due to disease, injury to the scalp and unwise or excessive use of hair cosmetics and dry weather.

The reason why so many adolescents have dandruff is that this is the time when they secrete an excess of androgen hormones which cause sebum, the skin oil.

HOW TO GET RID OF DANDRUFF

The motto of hair-care is **keep it clean**. Wash your hair and scalp frequently—it could be daily or every other day depending upon how stubborn your dandruff is. If your hair and scalp are oily, you should use herbal shampoo, since washing hair with frequent strong shampoo can harm your hair.

Massage and daily brushing is extremely helpful in treating dandruff. They invigorate the blood circulation to scalp, promote the traffic of oil effusion and dislodge the dead skin cells sticking to the scalp for easy exfoliation. If you have dry dandruff, use an oil to massage your scalp especially before washing your hair.

Lastly, eat less animal fat, and more poly-unsaturated vegetable oils. Avoid nuts, chocolate, fried food, shellfish, iodized salt. Follow a diet high in greens, chicken, fish, milk and its products and food high in Vitamins A, E, and B Complex.

HOME–MADE COSMETIC CARE

Dandruff is one problem which can be easily taken care of with some home-made recipes.

FOR OILY DANDRUFF

Trifla Lotion

Buy some *trifla* from the market. Mix 1 teaspoon of it in one glass of water and boil. Let it simmer for about three minutes.

Cool it and strain it. Mix with equal quantities of cider vinegar or malt vinegar and massage the lotion in the scalp gently and leave it on. Use as a nightly massage. Shampoo with a mild shampoo in the morning.

Vinegar Rinse

To a mug of water, mix two tablespoons of malt vinegar. After shampoo, rinse the hair with it. Towel-dry your hair. This is an excellent remedy to prevent oily dandruff.

A Dandruff Cleanser

Soak two spoonful of fenugreek (*methi*) seeds in water overnight. In the morning, make a paste of the seeds and apply on the head. Leave it on for half an hour. Then wash the hair with soapnut (*Reetha*) or *Shikakai* and water. You may use a herbal shampoo instead to wash your hair. Do this routine twice a week.

FOR DRY DANDRUFF

Oil Massage

For best results, massage your scalp with 1 teaspoon hot castor oil, 1 teaspoon coconut oil and 1 teaspoon *til* oil. Leave it on for about half-an-hour and then shampoo it out. Follow this routine, twice a week, especially in winter.

Cleanser

Take about 5 tablespoons of yoghurt and squeeze half a lime in it. Take two spoons full of green grams and powder them. Mix it in curd. Apply on scalp and leave it for ten minutes. Wash your hair with a creamy shampoo thoroughly. Follow this routine at least once a week.

If the dandruff does not clear up in time, you should take medical advice. It could be due to a fungal infection.

Another effective dandruff chaser——A combination of a tablespoon of eau-de-cologne and two *aspirin* tablets crushed.

4

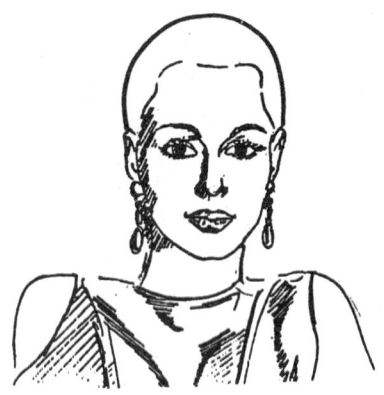

Dealing with Falling Hair

Hair, like human beings, has a life-cycle. Every hair that grows must fall out one day. New hair will grow at the same place, after some time.

There is a natural balance between the rate at which hair falls and the rate at which new hair grows. Any disturbance in this balance can result in an emotionally discomforting condition of either an excess fallout of hair or hairiness all over the body.

Now-a-days, excess loss of hair is very common. It happens for various reasons such as emotional and physical stress of city life, local scalp infection, adverse drug reaction, hormonal imbalances during teenage and pregnancy, etc.

FACTORS THAT DETERMINE HAIR LOSS

Over the past several years, dermatologists have made some interesting statistical findings that explain the pattern of hair loss. Curiously enough, the phenomenon of falling hair is provenly related to the rate of hair growth, length of the hair, age and even the colour of hair.

It is normal to shed from fifty to eighty strands of hair a day. It is normal for each of those hair to be replaced by the hard-working follicles. On any given day, about 90 per cent hair are in the growing stage. This period lasts for about 1000 days. Ten per cent hair are in the resting stage which lasts for about 100 days before the follicles eventually grow out.

Interestingly, the fall-out occurs mostly in the morning. This fact remains unexplained.

The length of hair is an important factor in hair loss. The four-inch long hair, loses on an average eighty seven hairs a day; the 12-inch long hair loses about twenty six hairs a day and 20-inch plus long hair loses as little as sixteen hairs a day on an average. *The longer the hair, the less is the hair loss.*

Hair grows on an average of 6 inches a year, and *shortfall in the normal hair growth is accompanied with a hair loss too.* Apart from the day-to-day loss, *we shed more than usual hair during six periods of our life*; from birth to age three; at ten, at twenty-two, around the age of twenty-six, at thirty six and around fifty-four. This happens due to hormonal changes that occur in our bodies during these periods of our lives.

The maximum hair growth on women occurs between the age of fifteen to thirty.

There are some other findings which the cosmetologists and dermatologists are currently investigating. It is felt that as and when these findings are credibly proven, the problem of hair loss would be better understood and its cure more possible.

CAUSES FOR THE EXCESS FALL OUT OF HAIR

Technically, an unnatural excess fall out of hair, temporary or permanent, is called *Alopecia* and is caused for reasons as explained.

Hereditary

The kind of hair we have—whether it is thick, thin, fine, sparse, straight or curly—depends a great deal on the genes inherited. The problems concerning hair loss are also passed on from the parents to the offspring. Diabetes and thyroid disorders are two real threats to healthy hair. Falling hair are also often directly inherited.

Trauma

The result of physical stress on the hair is called *Traction Alopecia*. This can be caused by tying up the hair in too tight *chignon* style, ponytails, or pigtails. The prolonged and continuing pull-like pressure on the hair can result in spot baldness.

Spot baldness is also caused due to a trauma or sudden shock experienced. A severe blow to the head may lead to spot baldness where the blow is received.

Local Scalp Infection

Bacterial, viral or fungal infections can cause spot fall out of hair. It can, however, be treated with medicated shampoos and lotions.

Diseases

Internal disorders and infections which cause high fever such as flu, pneumonia and typhoid are often accompanied by excessive hair loss.

Chemicals or Drugs

Antibiotics and a drug called *Cortizone* administered sometimes in treating acne and scars lead to hair loss. Chemical therapies given in serious diseases such as cancer, cause the excess fall out of hair.

Emotional or Environmental Stress

People unable to cope with pressures of life, all the time worrying about the problems at work place or home, having most of their emotional conflicts unresolved, are easy victims of excess hair loss.

With the tension in their minds, the muscles in the scalp and neck constrict. The blood circulation is thereby impeded, resulting in the suffocation of the hair follicles.

To prevent the consequential excess hair loss, massage to loosen up the scalp is an excellent remedy.

Hormonal Imbalances and Hair Loss

Hormonal imbalances are the primary cause of most serious hair loss conditions. Pregnancy, contraception with birth control pills and menopause are the common conditions that induce hormonal changes.

Pregnancy

Generally, the hair condition improves during pregnancy as the endocrine glands function at their peak.

The hair loss occurs only after the birth of the baby. This happens due to irregularity in the functioning of thyroid glands. It can be attributed to the change in the life style—the new unaccustomed life with the baby.

The normal hair loss after delivery happens four months after birth and continues for about two months.

Birth Control Pills

If a woman in perfect health with normal weight, having regular periods, eating sensibly and physically active, uses the pill for contraceptive reasons, she can expect the problem of hair loss. Taking the pill can alter her perfect hormonal balance.

In contrast if, however, a woman who is already suffering from hormonal imbalance takes the pill, it can restore the balance and promote hair growth.

Menopause

One of the problems of menopause is that the production of the female hormone *estrogen* slows down. This results in weak, dry hair and an excess fall out in one out of two women.

HOW TO PREVENT EXCESS FALL OUT OF HAIR

Hair in normal and healthy conditions does not fall out at an alarming rate. The excess fall out occurs mostly when the hair condition is extremely dry, rough and damaged.

Conditioning and nourishing of hair are the top priorities to prevent excess hair loss. Cream rinses help the dry and rough hair to regain its flexibility. Generous application of moisturisers and oil preparations replenish the moisture and oil in the dry hair.

Massage is a very important element of the scalp treatment to control excess fall out of hair. It invigorates the blood circulation, giving hair an increased supply of nutrition and oxygen for healthy growth. Massage also stimulates the dormant hair follicles to grow fresh hair.

THE HOME–MADE COSMETIC CARE

Try these age-old recipes.

The Hair Rejuvenating Ointment

Powder 10 gm each of lime seeds and black pepper. Make a fine paste in plain water or if possible in ginger juice. Apply this paste on the head every night. Leave it on for at least a couple of hours. Then rinse it out. Massage your scalp with your finger tips for five minutes while applying the paste.

The Magic Recipe to Treat Spot Baldness

- Make a paste with a few small sticks of *Mulathi* in milk cream. Add a little saffron and apply it on the bald patches at night. Rinse it out with clear water in the morning. If possible, mix some ground *Dhatura* seeds in the paste. It increases the potency of the recipe.

Massage your bald scalp spot generously with your finger tips for 5 minutes while applying the ointment.

The Wonderful Oil Massage

- Castor oil is excellent for hair re-growth. If combined with white iodine which is available at the chemist shop, it can produce the desired results.
- Part your hair in small sections and apply the oil to the scalp with cotton. Massage it in with your finger tips. If you are able to get white iodine solution, use it similarly on every alternate day.
- Squeeze the milk out of 1/2 a coconut, add the juice of half a lime and massage into the scalp. Leave on for 4 to 6 hrs. Wash with a mild shampoo or crushed *Hibiscus* leaves mixed with a tablespoon of crushed *fenugreek* seeds and made into a paste.

DO'S AND DON'TS

a. In case of baldness due to fungal, viral or bacterial infections, consult a dermatalogist.
b. Use a soft brush with well-spaced bristles.

c. Sanitise your implements, i.e. brushes, combs, etc. atleast once a week.
d. Drink a glass of carrot juice to which juice of half a lime has been added and 2 yeast tablets (*Brewer's yeast*).
e. Take iron tablets in case you are anaemic.
f. Improve the protein content of your diet.
g. Take birth control pills with a prescription.

The most important aspect of any treatment is the correct diagnosis. Unless it is well determined by observing the physical characteristics and studying the other causes for hair loss, the treatments given may not work efficaciously. It is advisable to seek professional help in cases of severe hair loss.

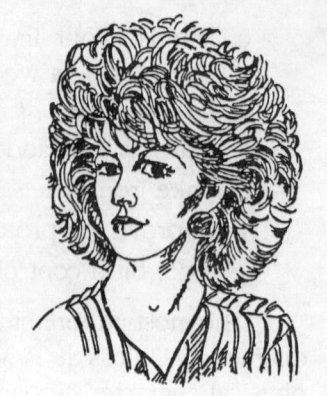

5

Colouring Your Hair

None of us wants to look older than our age and few of us welcome those first grey hairs. In fact there is no such thing as grey—only white colourless hair mixed with brown which gives an illusion of grey.

Grey hair on one's head does not necessarily mean advancing age. White hair can appear in the teens or twenties and there are a few lucky people who never go grey. But mostly white hair first begins to show in the thirties. The body just stops making colour pigment.

The process of oxidation haircoloring consists of:

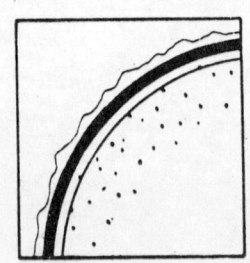

1. WETTING THE FIBER SURFACE WITH THE MIXTURE OF INTERMEDIATES IN A BASE WITH PEROXIDE, SWELLING THE HAIR FIBER, SIMULTANEOUSLY.

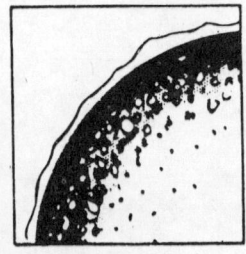

2. PENETRATION OF THE INTERMEDIATES ALONG WITH THE DEVELOPMENT OF COLOR.

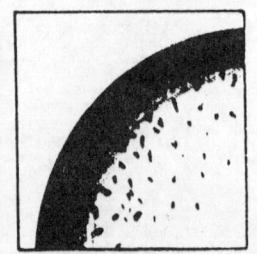

3. RINSING TO REMOVE UNREACTED INTERMEDIATES AND WEAKLY HELD SURFACE COLOR.

No one can go grey overnight. Even though shock or illness may affect production of pigment it is not until the new hair has grown that you see it is white.

Those of you who would prefer not to colour your hair, should choose softer colours in clothes and make-up, since the skin colouring is also toned down by the same natural ageing process.

White hair can be dry and wiry, so a conditioner is a must. Even the cleanest white hair can go yellow at the edges from smoke, dust and dirt in the hair.

To go further into the subject of colour, an understanding of the colouring treatment is essential.

TEMPORARY HAIR COLOURING RINSES

In this treatment, the hair shaft is coated with clear colour to darken or highlight. If you are not going to fight the white, the temporary rinse will keep it looking bright. It really is temporary, coating each hair only until the next shampoo. Colours come in coloured conditioning setting lotions, water rinses and shampoos, and will enhance white hair with silver pearl or blue colours.

A rinse can also add burnished gold or copper highlights to light or medium-coloured hair. It can bring out the red in the hair and brighten your dark hair with shine. With your next shampoo, the rinse washes away completely.

SEMI-PERMANENT TREATMENT

Shampoos of semi-permanent hair colourants come in one bottle and need no mixing. They penetrate the hair slightly and don't require the aid of a peroxide developer. The hair colour produced by such products fades gradually and naturally, lasting through four to six shampoos. As the colour fades, there is no root retouching to do. But most semis will only hide up to 25 per cent grey. They blend white hairs into your natural shade, but usually don't cover them completely. The secret of success is to choose a colour as near your own as possible. Semi-permanent colouring is rather easy to do on your own. The results are very natural-looking and the colour never rubs off on linen or clothing. Touches aren't necessary because a new application is repeated every four weeks.

HAIR COLOURING TREATMENT WITH CHEMICAL DYE

If you have a lot of white hairs, only a permanent colourant will cover them. Look for packs with two bottles to mix. One contains colour, the other peroxide which helps the colour penetrate deeply into the core of each hair to give longer lasting colour (six to eight weeks), and biggest colour change. You can even lighten your hair. Most are shampooed on. The colour doesn't wash out but after about every four weeks, the roots will need re-touching. Modern applicators make it easy to apply the colour just where you want on the roots where the new hair growth is showing.

The disadvantage of oxidation colouring is that it makes the hair dry and porous, so use plenty of conditioners. The hair colourants now available in the market are ammonia-free. Ammonia is a strong alkali used to make the colour compound penetrate deeply. But colourants formulated without it, are less likely to irritate the skin, do not smell so strongly and leave the hair in better condition.

Today there are two kinds of permanent hair colouring products available; penetrating tints and coating tints, like herbal hair dyes.

The subtlest way of camouflaging grey hair is to have streaks done professionally. Tiny, thread-like sections of hair are tinted all over the head, and as hair is made up of several

Colouring Your Hair

different shades, results can be very natural-looking. Less retouching is necessary.

COLOURING HAIR AT HOME

Henna

Different shades are made by mixing *Henna* powder with the following: *Henna* powder 2 cups, warm water 1 cup, lime juice 1 teaspoon. Stir *henna* powder and water into a thick paste. Add lime juice to help release the dye. Let stand for one hour.

One or more tablespoons of ground cloves mixed with *henna* will get a darker shade.

A dark brown shade may be obtained by mixing one part *henna* to 3 parts indigo.

A tablespoon of coffee and 2 tablespoons *amla* powder mixed with henna also darken the resulting shade.

To counteract the drying action add curd and a tablespoon of raw mustard oil.

Walnut Shells

Walnut shells make another harmless dye which progressively adds colour to the hair. Put walnut shells in a mortar and cover with water. Add a touch of table salt. Let it stand for 3 days. Now add 3 cups of boiling water and simmer for 5 hours, always making sure that the evaporated water is replaced. Express the dark liquid from the shells by means of a press or by twisting the shells in a cloth. Replace separated liquid in the pot again and now reduce to a quarter of its volume. Add a small piece of alum as fixative. At first it will produce a somewhat yellowish effect, but it will finally give the hair a good deep black colour. Remember to use on clean shampooed hair.

Boil 4 teaspoons of any tea in a quart of water until a

very dark brown liquid is obtained. Alum is used to set the dye. Strain and use like a rinse. Repeat rinses until the desired shade is acquired.

HOW TO CHOOSE A COLOUR

Now you know the methods you can use to change the colour of your hair, but the most important point is determining the colour that's correct for you. You can't just make a blanket statement and say "I want my hair to look the way it did when I was twenty-five." When you were twenty-five, your dark hair looked right with your complexion. A quarter of a century later, however, that same near-black hair will be much too harsh for your skin and face and will, in fact make you look older.

The rule to follow is the darker your hair colour, the younger you should be. The older you are, the lighter your hair colouring should be.

HOW OFTEN TO COLOUR HAIR

The primary rule is, avoid overlapping of colour by retouching surfaces every four weeks. No more and no less. Exactly every four weeks. If dyeing or bleaching is scheduled sooner, you overprocess the previously treated hair and this is very noticeable from the hair's dry and brittle appearance. If you colour or bleach five or six weeks later, you underlap the previously treated hair and create an uneven structure of the hair.

This is harmful since the original chemical process of dyeing or bleaching alters the structure of the hair to begin with. So an exact four-week retouch is a must.

In addition, after colouring, you must allow your hair to remain dry for three days and three nights to allow the process to oxide properly.

RULES TO REMEMBER FOR AT-HOME COLOURING

1. **Always do a patch test.** This is extremely important, especially when you are using a market product for the first time. Use a cotton ball to remove any natural oil from behind your ear or in the crook of your elbow and then apply a dab of the colouring product. If, within 24 hours, you experience any breaking out or itching, take an antihistamine (Avil is fine), drink plenty of liquids, wash the experimental area off well, and throw out the stuff! Don't skip this important patch test: allergic reactions can be devastating.

2. **Work with dirty hair.** Always use hair colour or bleach on hair in its soiled state. It's a mistake to shampoo it first, contrary to directions on most do-it-yourself products. The oil actually protects the skin against the unwanted invasion of chemicals into the system. In fact, the morning before colouring your hair, don't even brush it.

3. **Don't fight the red in your hair.** Amateur colourists make the mistake of trying to eliminate any red pigmentation. But red pigment is an important factor in the actual structure of the hair. If you try to remove this colour via overtinting or bleaching, you remove the last link that holds the chain reaction of the hair itself together. And especially to dark hair, more red highlights are good and flattering, so exploit them, don't eliminate them.

6

Selecting Hair Style

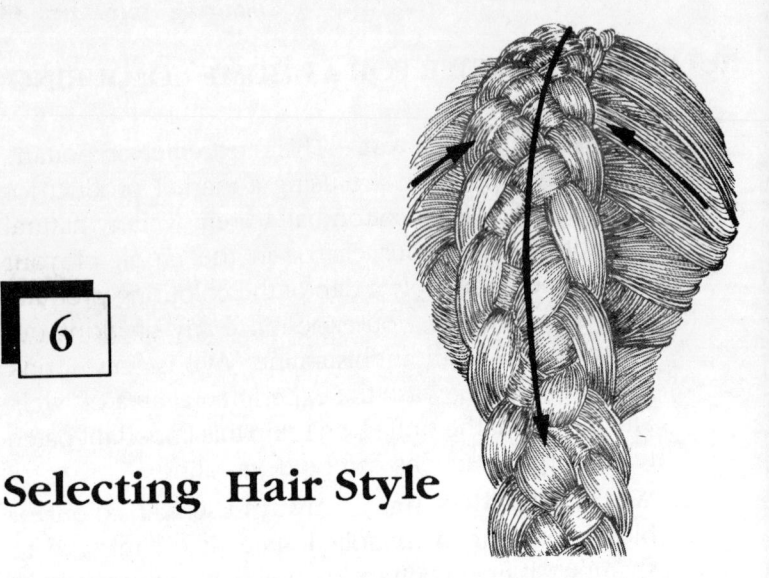

In hairstyling, there is no such thing as "one style fits all". Every woman is unique and special in her looks. A hairstyle is designed to befit the face shape, body, relate to the lifestyle and more.

While selecting your hairstyle, there are a few principles to remember. They can help you to choose a style that is more becoming for you.

HEAD SHAPES

Hair designers are often asked questions about head shapes and their proportions to hairstyling. Keeping in mind the below mentioned relationship to body height and styles, the following considerations can give the illusion of the classic oval shape face.

Generally, height or fullness is added to areas that fall short. Closeness is created where the arc is extended. In this manner, a balanced look is achieved. It is important to increase or decrease the right amount of hair needed to create the proper hair-face relationship and to adapt the hairstyle to the general shape.

STYLE AND BALANCE

Keep in mind that the normal proportion of head size to total height is measured at $7^1/_2$ heads of height. Regardless of height, the head can be put in proportion with the body by controlling the size of the head form. Whatever the fashion mode of the day, hair should reflect its proper proportion in relationship to the body. To achieve the proper form, consideration must be given to the density, texture, and weight of the hair and the process it must undergo.

WHAT TO LOOK FOR IN A HAIRSTYLE

Although only you, with your individual taste and preference can dictate the style you want, a consultation with your professional hairstylist is highly recommended. However, the finished product should be attractive, healthy looking and easy to care for.

Triangular Face: The triangular face usually displays a jaw line that is somewhat pointed. In order to balance and detract, widen silhouette in symmetrical (balanced) form, and ease more hair onto the face to correct the irregularity.

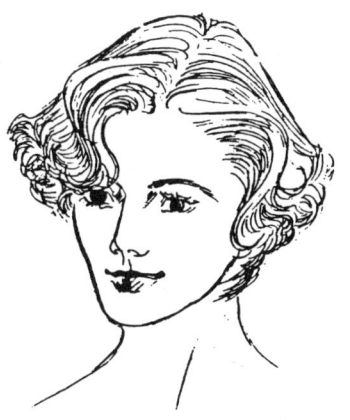

Square Face: If the face or jaw is square, add height in the centre of the style to minimize the squareness. Add slight width to further narrow the jaw. This also eliminates any chance of a square silhouette in the upper part of the style.

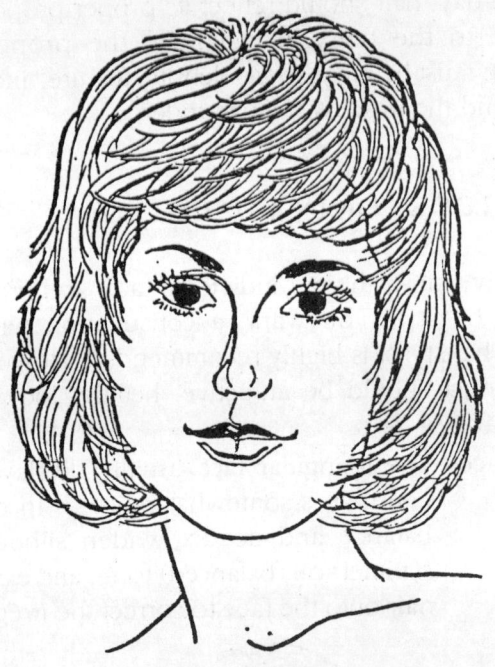

Long Face: In dealing with length in the facial structure asymmetry (unbalanced form) will detract from the length of the face when the line of vision moves horizontally rather than vertically. Do not add height, but do add some hair on the forehead to aid in creating a pleasing shape.

Round Face: A round face can be improved by moving hair on the face to break the round hairline growth. Hair on the forehead should move horizontally to contrast the rounded

Selecting Hair Style 37

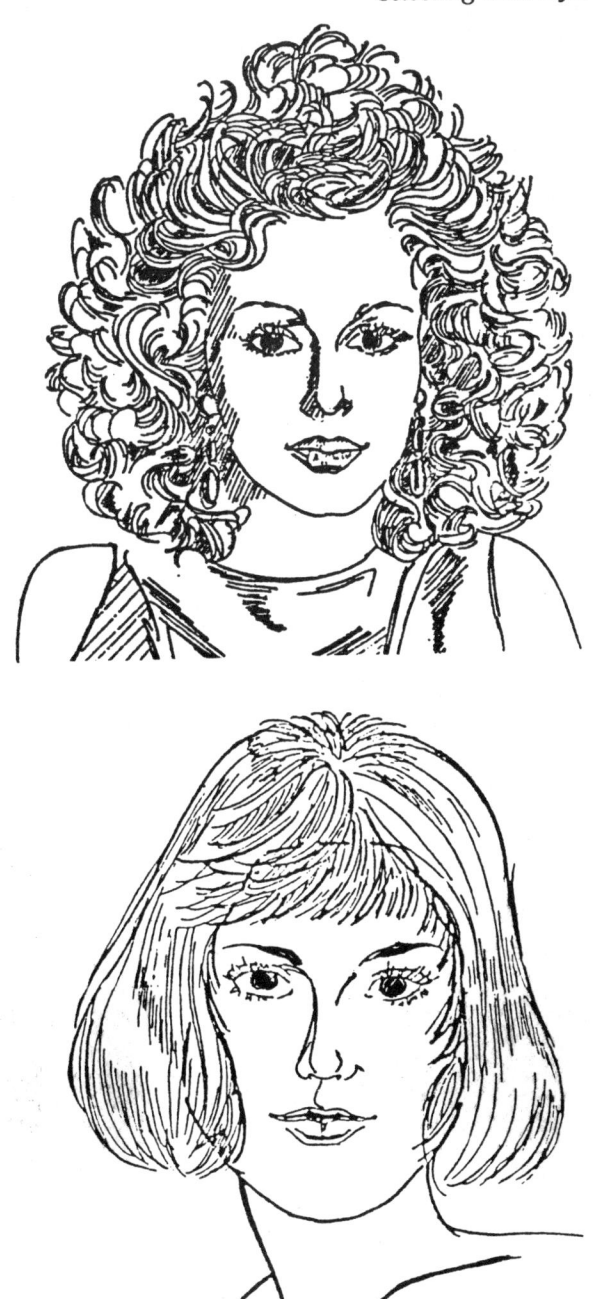

chin line. Asymmetry (lack of balance) in form, creates horizontal lines to contrast roundness.

It is with the aid of proper cosmetics and through the careful placement and proportion of hair fashions that facial irregularities are minimized and do not become dominant characteristics.

Every face has some imperfections. The best part is that most of these imperfections can be corrected by styling your hair well. Here are a few suggestions to deal with some of the common irregularities of the face.

Receding Forehead and Chin

If the forehead and chin recede, fullness over the forehead creates balance with the nose line and conceals the extreme slope.

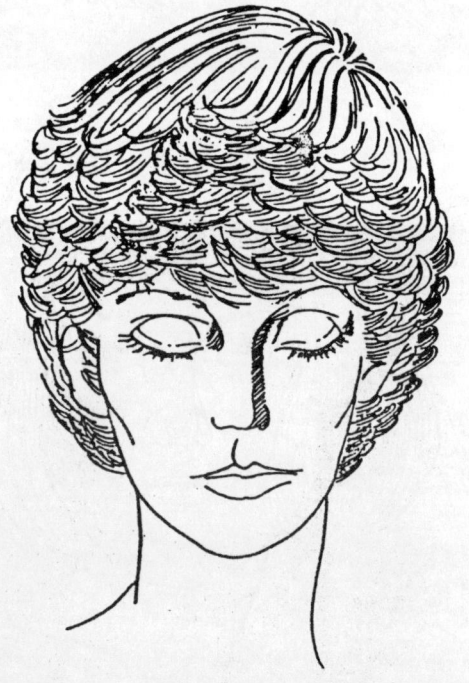

Long Jaw Line

If the jaw line is long creating a great deal of facial area, it must be balanced with the proper positioning of the hair. Lower the side-hair motions on to the face to decrease the facial area in view.

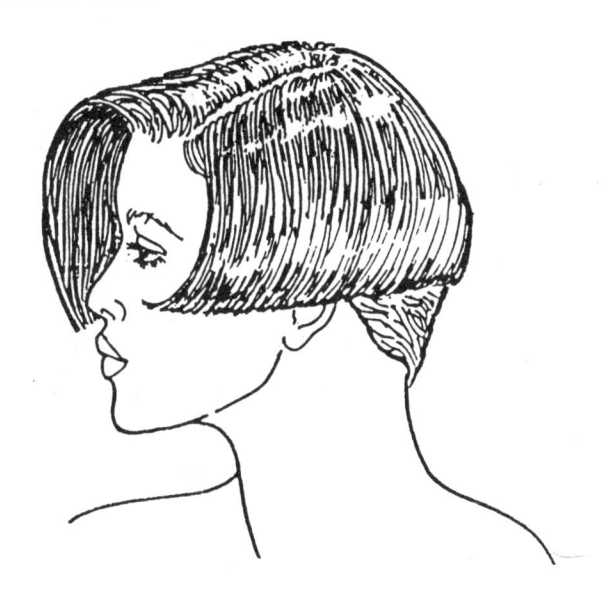

Low or Small Forehead

Design a style with hair off the face and create height in the style. A short hair-cut in front will give the forehead a higher look.

Ears that Stick out

Avoid a short hair style. Design hair that slightly covers the ears and masks the problem entirely.

In creating a hairstyle, it is important to remember the objective, i.e. to ovalise the face shape.

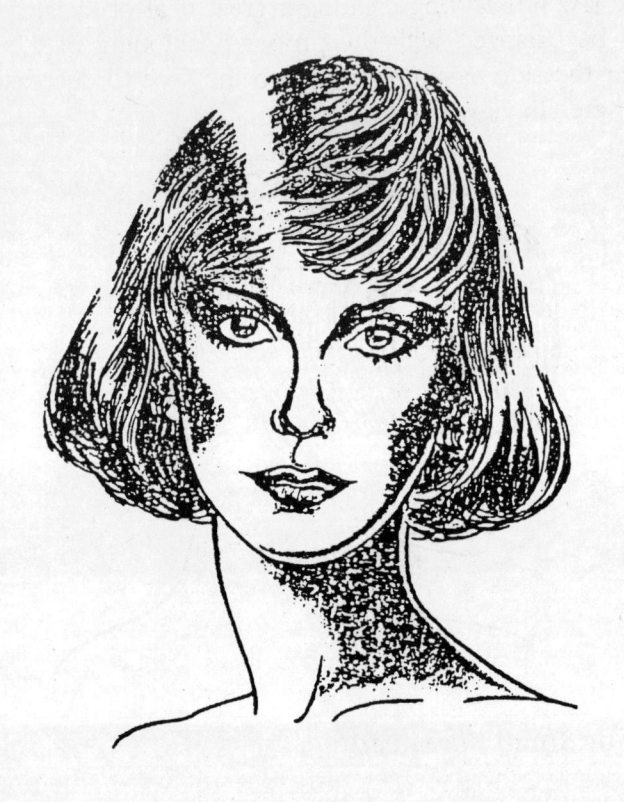

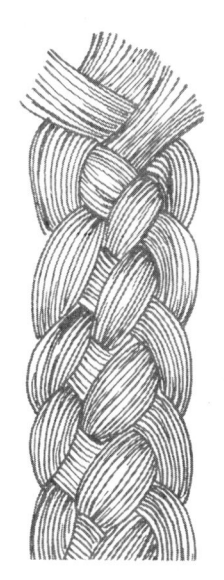

7

Caring for Long Hair

Shining long hair, flowing loose or carefully dressed remains a sure symbol of feminity even in this age of change and controversy. Some experts believe women let their hair grow to flaunt their beauty and their sex-appeal.

Long hair needs special care and when long hair isn't properly cared for, it begins to look like a rope left outdoors for months.

Shampooing with the correct shampoo, specially formulated for long hair is very essential. After shampooing your hair, take care as wet hair is very fragile and can break easily.

After washing your hair, don't brush instantly. Wrap it in a towel and blot out some of the moisture. Rubbing splits the ends and tugging very wet hair in its weakened state, pulls out the hair. When your hair is slightly dry, comb it with a wide toothed comb, starting from the ends slowly working up to the crown. In this way you avoid tangles and excess pulling.

A problem faced by many is, oily scalp, coupled with dry and split ends. Follow your shampoo with a final rinse of diluted vinegar—one tablespoon of vinegar to a mug of water. This helps restore the acid mantle that has just been washed away. Also, use a good creamy conditioner only on the ends.

Oily hair also requires brushing to keep oil from pooling on the scalp and to carry the oil to hair ends to prevent the ends from drying out and splitting.

Correct brushing with the correct brush is probably the single most important factor in long hair-care. Use a brush with natural bristles or with rounded synthetic bristles set in a back that is durable with a handle which fits comfortably in your hands. The best way to brush your hair, of course, is with your head hung down, while you brush finely from nape to ends of hair and all round. Use firm, even strokes. Don't tear your hair and don't yank it.

Leading trichologists recommend frequent massage of the scalp. Massage, certainly loosens the scalp and improves the circulation, giving elasticity to the hair. Start massaging with the fingers together at the top of your head using the cushions, not the tip of your fingers. Make rotary movements, working over the entire scalp and moving the scalp, not the fingers.

Split ends especially in long hair are a result of rough treatment of your hair. Fierce brushing snaps the hair and breaks it off. The use of rubber bands to tie hair together, and winding hair into a fish hook with metal curlers or rollers can damage your long tresses. To avoid split ends, your hair deserves gentle, capable handling. First trim the hair off above the split. Keep them under control by using a cream conditioner on the dry ends. Don't use metal or wire rollers.

Girls who wear long hair in tight plaits and women who wear a tight chignon seems to be the most frequent victims of spot baldness. It is caused by pulling the hair tightly back in an elastic band or bun in exactly the same place for a long period. The position of a pony tail or a bun and the parting of these hair-dos should be changed often if loss of hair is to be avoided. Hair pulled back into confined styles should have the benefit of extra care in correct brushing and massage.

Once again, those of you who use electric rollers, curling irons and blow dryers, be sure to condition your hair after shampoo and use hot oil treatments regularly to keep hair from drying out.

Caring for Long Hair 43

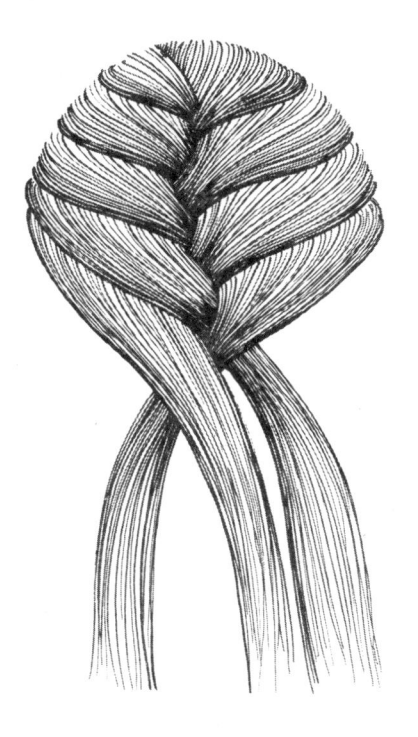

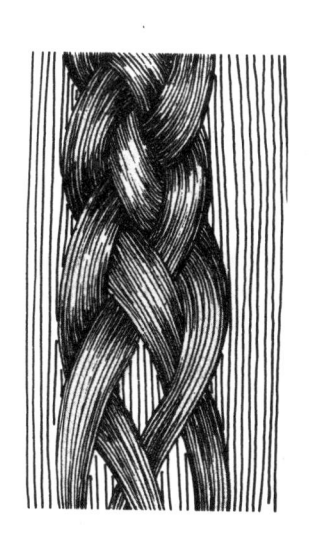

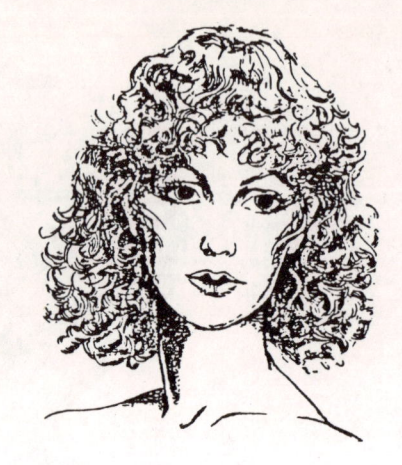

Perming Hair

Today's new perms are professionally designed for the active, on-the-go lifestyle.

There is a special perm for every individual, depending on the texture, condition and style of the hair. Every perm can and should be as individual as your own hairstyle and lifestyle.

Any perm can give you curls, but successful restructuring of the hair necessitates the expertise of a professional cosmetologist. Their knowledge and experience is essential in determining exactly what technique is required to create the look designed just for you.

The advantages of permed hair are numerous. The finished perm offers the wearer adaptability and versatility. The hair benefits from the support of a professional body wave, both aesthetically and functionally.

HOW OFTEN SHOULD ONE HAVE A PERM ?

As the name implies, curl is permanently waved in the hair. Although the curl may relax a little after shampooing and day-to-day wear, it will never entirely go away. As the hair grows and you have your hair cut, your perm will be cut off. The new growth from the scalp will be straight and on the average, most people need a new perm every 3 to 4 months. When your hair does not hold the style you desire, lacks body, then it is time for a perm.

THE DIFFERENCE BETWEEN A SALON AND A HOME PERM

A salon perm is different from a home perm in that most perm lotions contain chemicals that damage hair when used by inexperienced users and frequently result in under-processing—that is little or no wave. Your stylist, however, has the technical knowledge and expertise to know exactly which strength of perm solution, rod size, and wrapping technique is best for your hair and hairstyle. Your stylist's technical training and professional knowledge also allows him/her to select the proper timing for the curl reformation.

HOW LONG DOES THE SERVICE TAKE ?

With today's busy lifestyles, the busy woman is hesitant to allow time for a perm. Once the decision is made to have a perm, allow from $1\frac{1}{2}$ to $2\frac{1}{2}$ hours for the service. The largest part of the service and one of the most important is the wrapping of the hair on the perm rods. Do not try to rush your stylist; some wrapping techniques can take as long as one hour.

WHAT ABOUT PRICES ?

The price of a salon perm varies just as the price of a hair-cut does, depending on the salon, stylist, condition of your hair and the style you want. Whatever be the price, this is a small price to pay for an important fashion accessory that you wear 24 hours every day.

WHEN SHOULD ONE HAVE A HAIR-CUT, BEFORE OR AFTER ?

Hair can be cut before the perm, after the perm or not at all. This depends on your stylist, your personal style preference and the condition of your hair. Your professional stylist will be glad to advise you.

DOES NATURAL CURLY HAIR REQUIRE A PERMANENT WAVE ?

People with curly hair do get perms, to re-direct the natural curl into a more manageable pattern or to achieve a particular look or style and to even out the curl. Also if you would prefer a smoother, less curly look, a perm on larger rods can reform the curl into a larger smoother curl pattern. Your professional cosmetologist is trained to redirect your curl pattern the way you want it to be.

SOME CAUTIONS ON PERMANENTS

1. There is no reason why anyone cannot have a perm. However, if you have skin abrasiveness or scalp irritation, it is advisable to tell your stylist and wait until they are healed before proceeding with the service.
2. Some medications build up on the hair shaft affecting the results of the perm.
3. Some people who have abused their hair will need a series of treatments prior to a perm service; and
4. Always consult your professional cosmetologist who will advise you about the proper procedures.

9

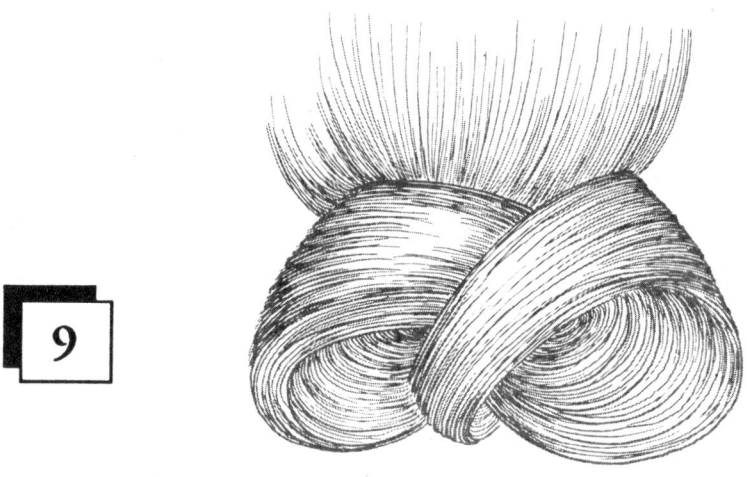

Managing Your Hair

Every woman needs hair that is neat, simple, flattering and easy to maintain. To end up with this kind of hair, you have got to begin with the right hair-care tools and a practical manageable style.

HAIR CARE CHECKLIST

Caring for your hair will be much simpler if you have got the right products for your particular hair type as well as styling equipment that really performs. Here's a checklist to follow.

Shampoo

A good shampoo is the number one item, or better still, make it several good shampoos. Although manufacturers insist that you don't need to switch shampoos (at least not away from their brand), as the weather and the condition of your hair changes, you may certainly want to change from brand to brand.

The best shampoo is not the most expensive, the one with the normal PH or the most enchanting scent. It's the one that works best on your hair. Ask friends or your hairdresser for recommendations and don't be afraid to try new products to find those that work best for you.

When you have found it, decide just how often your hair must be washed to look its best. If your hair needs everyday care, don't try to get by with washing it every other day. No matter how good the cut or how pretty the style, your hair can't look its best if it isn't clean, fluffy and manageable. (If you do have to shampoo frequently, keep the style as simple as possible so you don't feel as though you're spending all your free time on your hair).

Conditioner

Hair that's washed frequently, permed or coloured, or regularly exposed to heated hair appliances, will probably need a conditioner. Choose an instant liquid conditioner to apply after each shampoo. Once a month, treat your hair and scalp to a deep conditioning treatment for extra nourishment. If your hair is damaged, use the deep conditioner more often, say, two or three times a month.

Also remember that if the hair is really damaged, a conditioner cannot *cure* it, only make it look and feel better. To achieve a head of healthy hair, you've got to cut off the damaged parts and start all over again.

Blow-Dryer

These come in all sizes and wattages, some with the styling equipment, some solo. The one that's best for you is the one you find easiest to use with good results. (If you must travel for your job, invest in a small blow-dryer that's easy to pack).

Curling Iron

It is rather time-consuming to create a complete style with a curling iron but this appliance is great for touchups or a few quick curls. You might keep a portable curling iron ready in your purse or desk drawer for reviving a wilted hairstyle.

Brushes and Combs

For just plain brushing, choose a brush with natural bristles or one with heavy plastic bristles embedded in a rubber cushion. If you like nylon bristles, be sure you check to see that the tips are rounded. Any bristles cut straight across can tear your hair.

When you blow-dry your hair, you will want a round, natural-bristles brush. These come in several sizes—the larger brushes create a fuller, looser style; smaller ones are best for a tighter, curlier look. The easiest comb to use is one with a handle or "Tail". Pocket combs work only for very short hair.

Setting Tools

If electric appliances don't do the job for your hair, you do have other options. Rollers, either the foam kind or hard plastic ones, will give you a full, fluffy style. Stay away from brush rollers or rollers secured with hair picks as they both tend to break hair. Bobby pins or clips can be used for pin curls which produce effects, ranging from deep waves to fine ripples.

Setting Aids

If you do set your hair with rollers or pin curls, save time with setting gels and lotions. You can put more hair on each roller, if you take advantage of these setting aids and your style will also last longer. After the comb-out, hair spray will help to hold the line of your style but be careful not to overspray.

Hair Accessories

Try plain barrettes or small hair combs to rescue a fallen style. If hair is longer, you can sweep it back with a coated band. Have a ready supply of these in your make-up bag or desk drawer for when your hair–or the weather–has an off day.

CHOOSING A HAIRDRESSER

A good hairdresser is just as vital to pretty hair as the right hair-care equipment and the ideal style. However, a good hairdresser is hard to find. Here are some tips to help you in your search.

Your hairdresser should give you a style that fits both your hair-type and your lifestyle. If you spend a great deal of time outdoors, on the job or off, you don't want a hairstyle that must be constantly protected from the weather elements.

The same goes if you live in a damp or windy climate. Don't let anyone talk you into a difficult style.

You must be able to manage your hair yourself between visits to the salon. Does your style look good only after it's been professionally done? Then it may be time to find a new hairdresser who's a better stylist.

The cut should grow out gracefully, too. If it is scruffy and scraggy by the third week, the cut wasn't good to begin with. Even hair that grows rapidly should look good for about five to six weeks.

One of the best ways to find a good hairdresser is through word of mouth. (Trial and error works but the errors can be very trying). So ask friends, neighbours, co-workers, even strangers whose hair-dos you like, for the name of their hairdresser. It's detective work that should pay off.

THE SKIN SECTION

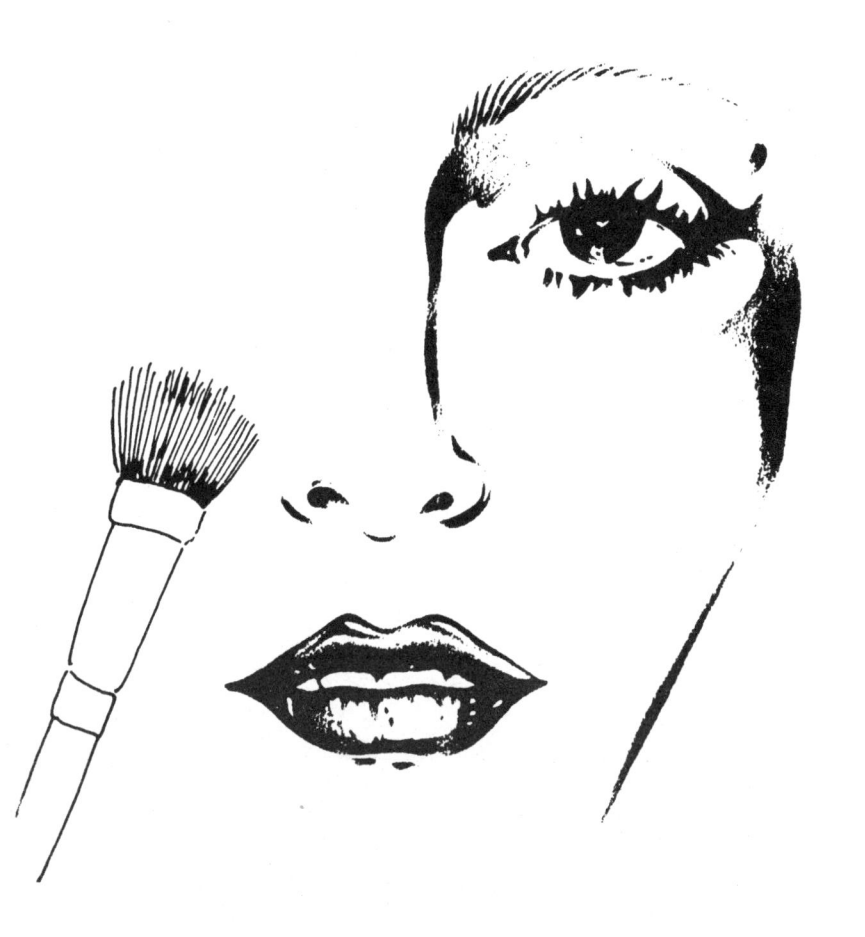

10

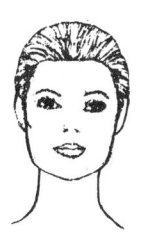

Understanding the Skin and its Care

Our skin is, perhaps, the most vulnerable organ in the body. It is constantly exposed to the pollution, grime, and the adversities of the weather conditions. Not surprisingly, skin problems are a common occurrence, and afflict almost everyone at some stage of their lives.

Good skin-care begins from day one. Not only does a neglected skin fade quickly and smell unpleasant as we all know, but also because the pores are clogged, it cannot perform its functions such as nourishment and purification properly—with the result that lack of care leads to disturbance in the body system. So get to know your skin. In order to understand and deal with common skin problems at home, and also to follow an effective day-to-day skin-care, it is important to first understand skin—its structure and its functions. Here is a brief summary.

THE STRUCTURE OF THE SKIN

Our skin comprises three layers—the *epidermis*, the *dermis* and the *hypodermis*.

The outer layer is the *epidermis*—the part we see and touch. It is composed of dead horny cells formed by the protein *keratin* and a basal cell layer underneath where the new cells are manufactured. The new cells move upwards to the surface where they expire and then are exfoliated. Melanin cells which are responsible for freckles and darkening the skin's colour due to the ultraviolet rays in sunlight are also in the dermis. The epidermis has no blood vessels or nerves.

The *dermis* is commonly known as the true skin. It is made up of connective tissues which include collagen protein and elastic fibers (elastic-type protein) which form a valuable support system to the skin. It is in this layer that the majority of the skin's aging process takes place. The sweat glands, the oil glands, the nerve endings and receptors, blood vessels, *arrector pili* muscles and a major portion of hair follicles are also located in the dermis.

The *hypodermis* or *sub-dermis* is a subcutaneous tissue or fatty layer situated below the dermis. It influences the quality of our skin's appearance. A dramatic loss of weight causes the skin to sag and too much fat or water retention in the skin's tissue makes the skin stretch and dimple. The hypodermis is a cushion for the skin. It acts as a shock-absorber to protect the bones and to help support the delicate structures, such as blood vessels, nerve endings and hair bulbs. The layer gives contour and shape to the body and acts as an emergency reservoir of food and water.

There are two sets of glands found in the dermis—the *sweat glands* and the *oil glands*. The sweat glands are employed in the elimination of the water-soluble cellular waste. The oil glands secrete oil which lubricates the skin surface. This prevents the skin from excessive dryness and chapping. Blockages, congestion, over activity or under activity of these two sets of glands are considered the primary causes of our numerous beauty problems.

FUNCTIONS OF THE SKIN

Protection

The general perception is that skin is only a protective covering on the body. It is important to realise that the skin performs six other vital functions alongwith the protection it provides to the internal organs.

Elimination of Waste

It helps in eliminating the toxic waste products and water from the body. Poor elimination leads to sallow and dull complexion, swelling all over the body and aggravation of acne.

Regulation

It regulates the body temperature. Whatever be the temperature outside, it maintains its inside temperature.

Respiration

To a small extent the skin breathes, exhaling carbon dioxide and eliminating other unwanted gases.

Absorption

The skin permits certain substances to pass through its tissues.

Hydration

Maintains the moisture level of the skin by discharging perspiration and the oily sebaceous material that is the skin's best lubricant.

Sensation

The nerve ending under the skin makes us aware of heat, cold, pain and pleasurable sensations. Sensation helps us to react.

THE CHARACTERISTICS OF A HEALTHY SKIN

There are a host of features accredited to a healthy skin. The features help to recognise, and assess the condition of the skin.

In our common language (and the cosmetologist's lingo), a healthy skin condition is blemish free, (unpigmented, scar-free), soft and moist (not oily and not dehydrated), smooth and glowing (reflecting light and with clear visibility of the inner skin), supple, firm, wrinkle-free (toned, elastic and collagen enriched) and having no visible acne or allergy (unsusceptible to infection).

CARE OF A HEALTHY SKIN

Ordinarily, a healthy skin needs minimal attention in terms of time and efforts to be spent for its care. However, an inadequate or improper care can run down and ruin a healthy skin. A regular skin-care regime and disipline are absolutely essential.

If you want your skin to look attractive and healthy, there are a few rules you must follow.

Internal care of a perfect complexion requires sensible diet, plenty of water, adequate sleep, moderate exercise, and a calm disposition. All these contribute to a soft, beautiful skin.

Diet

What you eat goes to your skin through the blood stream.

Food for a pretty skin includes fruit and vegetables, lean meat, dairy products, whole grain breads and cereals. Be moderate in your intake of sweets, chocolate, starches and greasy food and food to which you might be sensitive. If you break out into hives the day after you eat fish or prawns or in bumps when you've indulged in an orgy of chocolate, you know which food to restrict in your diet.

Drink plenty of liquids. Moisture is the key word in complexion beauty. It begins with six glasses of water a day, and as much additional liquid in the form of juices, milk and the like.

Sleep

Your skin revives itself when you sleep. Eight hours nightly, if possible ten, is not too much. This means eight or ten hours each night, not five hours one night and eleven the next.

Fresh Air and Exercise

Oxygen is vital to your skin and blood cells carrying both oxygen and nourishment are circulated to every part of your body including your skin. If you are continually breathing in stagnant stale air, you cannot expect your skin to look pink and glowing with good health. Deep breathing exercises are a beauty treatment in themselves especially when you are filling your lungs with pure fresh air.

A brisk half-hour daily walk can do you as much good as an expensive facial, especially if you are relaxed and dressed for the walk and above all enjoying the walk. You will return home with a glow in your cheeks and a sparkle in your eyes and your skin will tingle with vitality. Exercise revs up your circulation carrying oxygen to the skin.

Emotion

Your skin is an accurate barometer of your feelings. Fits of temper or bouts of depression may result in outbreaks of blemishes or rashes. Next time, you lose your temper count to ten.

Elimination

Establish regular elimination habits. Retained toxins show as poor colour, circles under the eyes or skin blemishes. A couple of figs or dates a day can help in daily elimination. An excellent antidote to constipation is an early-morning drink of lemon juice and water, or a teaspoon of Malt vinegar and a tablespoon of honey stirred into a glass of hot water. Soak the dates overnight in a cup of water. In the morning, mash the dates in the water and drink first thing in the morning before your bed tea.

SKIN-CARE REGIME

An effective skin-care regime which yeilds maximum benefit to the skin comprises the *cleansing, toning, moisturising* and *conditioning* routines.

The skin-care, of course, varies from one skin type to another and the relative emphasis of the various routines in it also differs.

Cleansing is the most important aspect of skin-care. It is undertaken primarily to remove the stale make-up, clean the skin pores and exfoliate the dead cells which otherwise cause blockages on the skin's surface.

The daily cleansing routine should be followed with toning. The *toning* exercise helps in the stimulation of the skin, pores and invigorates the blood circulation.

The *moisturising* and *conditioning* routines conclude the daily skin-care. Moisturising helps in keeping the moisture in the skin. The conditioning routine restores the acid balance on the skin and corrects other such imbalances.

MASSAGE

Massage is a very important part of skin-care. Throughout history, beautiful women have recognized the beneficial effects of a regular facial massage. When applying moisturiser in the morning or conditioner at night, take a little extra time to turn your beauty routine into a therapeutic massage treatment which will make you feel good, both mentally and physically.

Massage helps keep skin pores healthy and increases the action of the excretory glands, actually helping your skin to cleanse itself. Massage arouses tissues, perks up every little cell, and creates a tingling feeling of well-being.

As well as improving the circulation, correct massage relieves nervous tension by relaxing and so eases out fine lines. It also strengthens face and throat muscles and removes scaly, dead skin, leaving the skin smooth, firm and glowing.

In order to massage correctly, it helps to know a little about the facial muscles. The diagram below shows the structure of the neck and face-muscles and the direction of the main muscle flow.

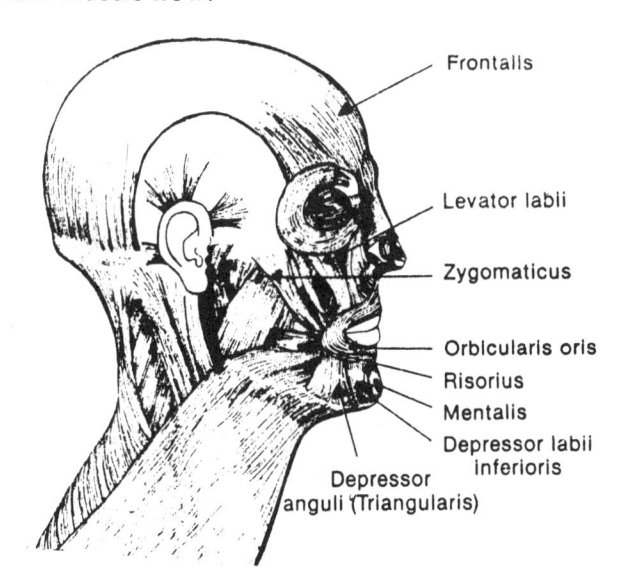

Most muscles flow in a general upward and outward direction which is why you should apply most face-creams in this way. It is important to massage in the direction that the muscles flow. Incorrect movements can pull muscles and cause them to sag. Be particularly careful to use a delicate movement near the eyes, where it is easy to stretch the skin and cause bagginess.

Facial Massage

- Massage for about 5 to 10 minutes daily or 20 minutes once a week.

    Using plenty of cream, start at the base of your throat. Massage from collar bone to chin tip and jaw bone one hand following the other in deep stroking movements. Do each movement 10 times.

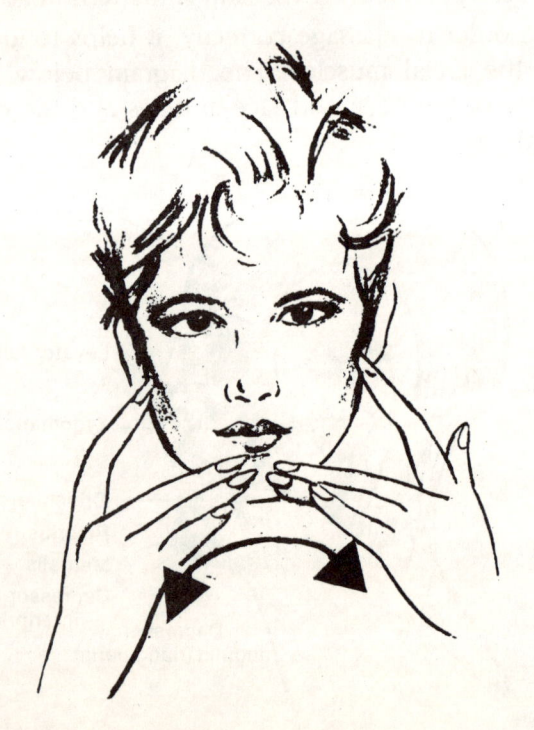

Understanding the Skin and its Care 61

- Using your index finger and thumb, *Pinch* or *Stroke* from your chin to the edge of your jawbone and back several times.
- Slap up under the chin with the backs of your hand. This helps circulation and reduces a double chin.
- Move on to treat your cheek muscles by working from your chin up across your cheeks to your temples with an *upward* and *outward* circling movement of your fingertips.
- Puff out cheeks. Pat with fingertips along the laugh line, from the corners of the mouth upto the nose.
  Massage your nose with small circular movements moving from the bridge of your nose to the nose tip.
- Massage under the eye from outer corners to inner corners and out over the eyelids. Using the second and third fingers sweep lightly out around your eyes in a gentle stroking movement from the bridge of your nose around to your temples, following the bone of your eye outside.
- *Play the piano* with quick little taps of your fingertips, moving from inner corners to outer corners, concentrating on little crows-feet at outside corners.
- To relieve tension, pinch your eyebrows, working from the bridge of your nose outwards. Make small circles at the temples.
- Using a brisk *scissor* movement of the first and second fingers, dance the tips horizontally up and over your forehead, starting at the centre and finishing at your temples. Using your ring and middle finger stroke up between the eyes and over the forehead finishing at your temples.
- There are two pressure points, one at the bridge of your nose where it meets your eye socket and the other at your temple just level with the end of your eyebrow. Gentle pressure applied at these points

with your fingertips and maintained for five seconds is very relaxing.

SKIN CONDITIONS

Every individual has a unique skin. Skin conditions can be generally characterised into three categories. Each person's skin can be related to one of the three.

Oily Skin Condition

It has a shiny appearance with large visible pores containing blackheads and whiteheads. The texture is thick, coarse and sallow yellow.

Dry Skin Condition

There are two types of dry skin conditions—the oil-dry and the moisture-dry. The oil-dry skin is sensitive and has flaky patches with no visible pores. It tends to age and wrinkles prematurely unless carefully looked after. The moisture-dry skin has a fine texture. Its appearance is taut and dry with a tendency to chap easily and even at an early age, may show tiny lines around the eyes and mouth.

Combination Skin Condition

It is a partly dry and partly oily skin. The central part of the face—the forehead, nose, chin and parts of the cheek—look glossy and oily. The other parts appear dry.

HOME-TEST FOR SKIN TYPE

The skin-type test: For the test, all that is needed is a few strips of tissue paper. Or you may use paper napkins instead.

In the morning, before washing your face, rub the strips gently across your forehead, nose, chin and cheeks by sliding them back and forth. The strips will either gain greasy stains or remain transparent and clean.

If the strips used on forehead, nose and chin are greasy, whereas the strips used on the cheeks are clean, you have a combination skin.

If all the strips are greasy, including the one used on the cheek, and the stains are large, you have an extremely oily skin.

If all the strips are clean and transparent it means you have a dry skin. Through the strip-test method, one can find out the skin-type and also which parts of the face and body are excessively oily or dry.

CAUSES FOR EXCESSIVE OILINESS AND DRYNESS

The oiliness is mainly caused due to the over-activity of the sebaceous glands and over-production of oil secretions. Alongside, if a proper cleansing routine is not followed, the condition worsens. The nervous and hormonal irregularities that occur in our bodies are presumably responsible for this over-activity of the oil glands.

Skin dryness is of two kinds: The oil-dryness is caused due to the sluggish activity of the oil glands resulting in inadequate oil secretions and an insufficient lubrication of the skin surface. Apart from the improper functioning of the sebaceous glands, jittery nervous conditions, improper diet, the use of wrong cosmetics, strong soaps, over-exposure to the sun and the harsh wind are some of the other factors that aggravate dryness.

The moisture-dryness is caused by the inadequate functioning of the sweat glands and internal dehydration. The natural elements such as sun and wind in extremes contribute to it. Increasing the liquids in diet and using skin moisturizers are extremely helpful.

The Beauty Complications

Oily skin looks greasy, unclean and aesthetically unappealing. The skin pores are visibly enlarged. Over a period of time, blockages of grime, stale make-up and horny dead cells appear in the skin pores, resulting in the formation of the unsightly whiteheads and blackheads.

The excessive oiliness engenders a sallow, yellow complexion and thick, coarse skin texture. The make-up alters and disappears easily.

The dry skin is thin and sensitive to weather elements and bacteria. It can develop an allergy easily. The skin usually tends to flake during the winters and fine wrinkles appear on the face prematurely.

The dark-coloured veins are obvious on the thin dry skin and the fine, red-coloured lines of the broken capillaries are also visible. The dry skin looks dull. Make-up tends to stand out and face powder looks floury.

SKIN CARE FOR OILY SKIN

Oily skin is the most painstaking and cumbersome to take care of. In order to treat an oily skin, it is important to carry out a scrupulous cleansing routine, sloughing off the dead cells, removal of stale make-up, excess oil and grime embedded in the pores.

The Cleansing Routine

Involves washing the face and neck at least twice a day with a mild, medicated soap. Avoid using creamy and fat-enriched beauty soap for washing the face. Concentrate on the forehead, nose and chin area. Massage the lather thoroughly. Rinse with clear cold water.

During the day, clean your face several times with cotton

saturated with a freshner or cleansing lotion. Toning and tightening the enlarged pores with an astringent is advised after cleansing the skin.

After using the toner, if the skin feels taut and dry, apply a mild moisturizer, which will not block or irritate the skin pores.

THE HOME-MADE COSMETIC CARE

Cleansing Scrub

Mix 1/4 cup *Multani Mitti* (fuller's earth), 1/4 cup dried orange peel, and 2 tablespoon sandalwood powder/oatmeal and store in a container in the bathroom. Take one teaspoon mixed with water and work it into the skin, rinse it with warm water. Use every other day.

Cleansing Mask

Mix 1/4 teaspoon fuller's earth, some tomato pulp and yoghurt in a little cucumber juice and apply on face for 15–20 minutes. Rinse it off with cold water. You should apply this mask atleast twice a week.

Toners

Mix a tablespoon of lemon juice or a tablespoon of malt vinegar in a glass of water.

Cabbage or cucumber juice, mixed with rose water are excellent toners as well. Add a pinch of alum and two drops of *spirit of camphor*. Keep a bottle of any of these toners handy for frequent use during the day.

Toning Mask

Make a paste of one beaten egg white, 1 tablespoon yoghurt and *multani mitti* (fuller's earth) and apply on the face till it dries. Later rinse off with clear water. Use this toning mask atleast twice a week.

Some Tips

- Avoid using cream or oil-based make-up products. Use only water-based cosmetic creams and powder make-up.
- Since the face has to be cleaned several times a day, use minimum make-up.

SKIN CARE FOR DRY SKIN

The dry skin is either oil or moisture-dry. The skin-care regime should emphasize the moisturizing and nourishing routines. The dry sensitive skin should be cleansed with a cold cream and alcohol-free skin fresheners to remove the cream.

After cleansing, the skin needs a lubricating emollient or a moisturizer. For best results, the moisturizer should be used while the face is damp after the wash.

THE HOME-MADE COSMETIC CARE

Dry Skin Cleanser

Warmed milk cures roughened skin. It can be added to oat meal, or almonds

Try this milk lotion. Warm a cup of milk and add 1 tsp. glycerine, 1/4 teaspoon bicarbonate of soda and 1/4 teaspoon borax till all three dissolve.

Melt together in a bowl, 12 tablespoons white vaseline (petroleum jelly), 4 tablespoons baby oil and 1 tablespoon bees wax. When heated, remove from fire. Add a few drops of rose essence and store in a jar and use to clean face. Remove the cleanser with a damp cotton.

Moisturiser

Mix 3/4 cup of rose water, 1/4 cup of glycerine, 1 teaspoon. of vinegar and 1/4 teaspoon of honey and keep it in a bottle. Use it regularly after cleansing.

Nourishing Mask

Mash a banana and beat in a teaspoon of salad or vegetable oil. Brush it on to the face and leave it on for twenty minutes till it dries. Then rinse it off. This nourishing mask should be used once a week atleast.

Some Tips

- Do not use an astringent or a toner containing alcochol.
- Avoid the sun and harsh winds and hot baths.
- Use oil-based creams and make-up products only.
- Do not use medicated soap. Use creamy and soft beauty soaps.

AGING OF THE SKIN

The skin condition changes as we grow older. The horny, dead surface of the skin renews every three or four weeks till the twenties. In the mid-thirties and forties, the renewal process takes twice the time.

Changes occur in the complexion and the tone of the

skin. The complexion looks dull and the skin's tone (vitality) diminishes.

Here are some important facts on the aging of the skin.

- With age, the sweat and the oil glands decrease in number and size and become sluggish.
- While the entire mass of the body shrinks with age, the overlying skin remains the same in extent. The excess skin sags and creases in the form of wrinkles.
- As we grow old there is a breakdown of collagen which gives the skin its elasticity. The body fluids dry out and the bones and muscles lose tissue.
- Lastly, there is substantial decline in the number of blood vessels in the skin resulting in the slowing down of circulation. The skin becomes increasingly sensitive to the heat and cold.

Though these changes are not obvious to us from day to day, they occur everyday as we age.

However, a study of the skin condition of women belonging to four different age groups—adolescence, 20 to 35 years, 35 to 50 years and 50 years old can reveal significant and the obvious differences—the tell-tale story of age.

Adolescence

The skin is affected by the hormonal changes which lead to oiliness and an outburst of acne. The skin is otherwise supple and firm.

20 to 35 Years

During this age, women peak endocrinologically. This results in the over-activity of the sweat and the oil glands causing excessive perspiration and oiliness. Large pores accompany the acne and the oily skin condition. In several cases, the first wrinkles appear in this age.

35 to 50 Years

The skin glands become sluggish. The skin becomes thinner, loses its suppleness and dries out. The skin colour begins to change and no longer remains uniform. Pigmented spots appear on the skin. Broken capillaries and veins become noticeable.

50 Years

The skin looks mottled and gains about three different shades of colour. Wrinkles and creases show prominently. The skin becomes extremely dry. Dark brown spots appear at several places on the skin.

YOUR SKIN-CARE PROGRAMME DEPENDS ALSO ON YOUR AGE

Age One to Twelve

If you have normal skin and it has no dry spots or blackheads, there is no special problem. But you would be wrong to think that you can neglect your skin or have no need to take care of it. Always use a good soap and preferably soft water, morning and evening. Rinse several times to remove every last trace of soap and splash with cold water. Apply light moisturising baby lotion to protect the skin and keep it soft.

For Soft Water

Boil some water, let it stand (cool). Add a little *boric acid* and a little *friar's balsam (tincture of benzoin)*

Ultra-Violet Radiation

We have known for quite a while that all ultra-violet radiation is cumulative and that every hour of sunlight a person gets whether at age one, or fifty adds up. But we did not realise until fairly recently that an hour of radiation is far more damaging to a child than to an adult. Of course if you can stay out of the the sun for several years, your skin will recuperate to some extent. But the harm caused by any period of exposure can never be completely reversed. So children should be taught to use sunscreens.

Home-Made Sunscreens: Use *calamine lotion* and *baby lotion* (equal quantity) to which is added a pinch of *zinc oxide*, before your child goes into the sun.

An hour before your child goes into the sun—mix vinegar with *olive oil* in equal quantities and apply to the areas exposed, leave for an hour and then wash off with mild soap. This prevents sunburn.

Adolescence

Your skin needs scrupulous care during this period because the hormonal changes that take place in your body at and after puberty frequently lead to oily skin and acne.

A greasy skin is inclined to be shiny, with open pores and blackheads as a result of over-activity of the sebaceous glands. To fight against this excess, take certain precautions.

Wash your face in warm water using a non-alkaline soap. Nothing will do your skin more good than washing it twice a day. Spray it with soda water.

Use commercial brands of astringents and also natural astringents like cucumber, lemon or apple juice.

Use once a week a face-pack or face-mask of one beaten white of egg and a few drops of lemon. Keep it on for 15 minutes, then rinse with lukewarm water.

At Night

Remove your make-up with a liquid make-up remover, and finish cleansing with an astringent. Finally, wash with warm water and a non-alkaline soap.

In the Morning

After washing with soap and water, freshen your skin with a skin tonic having a small spirit content. Then apply a moisturising lotion specially formulated for oily skin or *calamine* lotion.

Twice a Week

Treat your skin to a cleansing treatment by using a friction wash that cleans clogged pores with abrasive action. Moisten your face and hands with warm water. Then put a teaspoon of cleansing granules in the palm, work them into a rich lather and apply to the face. Massage gently for a few seconds. Concentrate on clogged pores and blackhead areas. Rinse off thoroughly with warm water.

Acne

Acne is a sign of changes in hormonal level in the system which shows itself by inflammation at the mouth of the sebaceous glands producing spots.

Precautions to be taken

1. Avoid preparations which contain vaseline.
2. Choose non-alkaline soaps.
3. Avoid too highly spiced or starchy foods.

Nightly routine for acne: Remove your make-up with a liquid make-up remover. Wash with soap and water. Then apply an anti-acne cream and leave it on all night.

Morning routine for acne: Wipe your face with an anti-acne lotion. Let this lotion dry naturally. Use *calamine* lotion with 1 per cent *phenol* (ask your chemist to prepare it). Apply as a protective lotion.

Twenty to Thirty-five

This is the time when you peak endocrinologically (when you have reached your maximum hormone levels). Your oil glands and sweat glands are most active. Your sense of smell and taste are most acute. You are at your peak sexually.

Oily skin is an ongoing problem for a great many young women during their twenties and thirties. And as long as it persists, frequent washing with soap and water can be helpful along with a daily shampoo.

Acne, like oily skin, is a manifestation of this peak period of hormonal activity. But it may indicate slight hormonal imbalance when it goes on for long, and hormonal tests are useful in helping to pinpoint the exact cause. If the tests do show an imbalance, medication can be prescribed to correct this.

Large pores are another problem you are apt to see more of during these years because oily skin and acne both contribute to this condition. A large pore is nothing more than the skin surface outlet of a large (and more active) oil gland.

To Control Open Pores

Tomato juice and honey mixed and applied to the skin daily for ten minutes and then rinsed off helps open pores.

Exposure to sunlight is something else you have to be careful about. Remember this is a time when you probably spend more hours out of doors walking, swimming and such that you are likely to at any later period. So the amount of sun you get is bound to be considerable and you really have to zero in on protection. You are, after all, still in a very susceptible phase—a young phase. Use sunscreens and sun blocks regularly and generously.

Wrinkles first appear during this period. And in order to forestall them there are a few things you can do. Those who smoke should cut out cigarettes. Smoking causes lots of little lines on your upper lip and may even be linked to crow's feet although we do not have strong evidence on this yet.

For Crow's Feet

Breadcrumbs soaked in milk with a few drops of sweet almond oil can be wrapped in muslin and placed warm over your closed eyes. Crow's feet can be greatly reduced by applying the above compress.

Circles under the Eyes are Another Problem

An excellent and very simple remedy is to gently dab around your eyes with a pad of absorbent cotton, soaked in warm tea.

For the Eye Lids

Touch the lids with a drop of sweet almond oil. This keeps it supple and smooth.

For Eyes

Close your eyes often, blink frequently, give them eye-baths.

Thirty-five to Fifty

It is about now that your skin is getting thinner, less elastic. It is beginning to show changes in pigment. Colour is no longer uniform. You have little set groves on the upper lip, around your eyes, and on your forehead. But more than that, there is a gradual increase in skin surface area. It is rather like wearing a skin that is several sizes too big for your face.

Fifty–Plus

Your skin gets quite a mottled look as you get older. If you look at a young person's skin, it is a single shade. An older person's has at least three shades sometimes four, and there are brown spots that do not belong.

Once a week, apply a face-pack of the following recipe.

- To one teaspoonful of whipped cream, add a pinch of *alum* and a few drops of *lavender oil*. Keep this pack on for about 20 minutes then rinse with lukewarm water with three drops of *Tr. Benzoin*.

There is one very annoying problem that you gradually begin to be aware of—a gully and groove, in the cheek area between the lower eyelid and the nose. The skin above gets unbelievably thin and the skin near the nose gets thicker. It is very hard to correct this except with *replacement therapy, collagen, silicone* or the like.

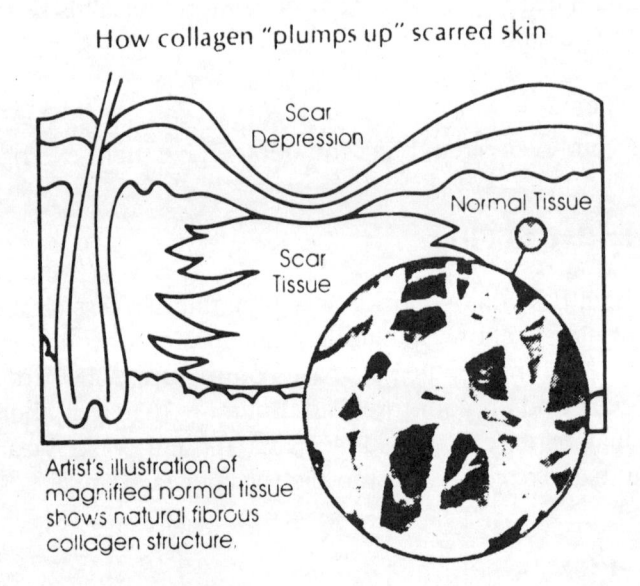

How collagen "plumps up" scarred skin

Artist's illustration of magnified normal tissue shows natural fibrous collagen structure.

Dry skin is more of a problem the older you get. As a woman's skin starts to get seriously dry, she usually tries to solve the problem by using just a standard moisturizer. She does not realise that skin-cell replacement has diminished as well as natural lubricant production. The key thing is getting the skin to be more the way it used to be. Exfoliation really helps. It sloughs off dead skin cells and also steps up cell division making skin cells perform more youthfully. You can get the cell division stepped up by tapping the skin and using an almond scrub. A large pinch of crushed almonds added to 1/4 teaspoon of your cleansing cream should be massaged well into the skin and rinsed off.

You can try the following masks.

- Separate the yolk from the white of an egg. Beat up the yolk with a little olive oil and spread the mixture evenly all over your face and neck. Leave it on for quarter of an hour. Remove it with lukewarm water.

Note: Never use warm water as that would set the yolk. Use almond oil with a few drops of essential oil of patcholi, morning and night (to maintain the rhythm of cellular reproduction) and then apply a moisturiser.

SOME INTERESTING FACTS

- The skin is the largest organ in the body.
- The skin of an average adult weighs about three kilograms and covers a surface area of sixteen to twenty square feet.
- A square inch of skin contains nearly 12 million living cells, 60 oil glands, 400 sweat glands, controlled by 4 sense organs each with 15 yards of nerve strands, 1200 sensory cells, 100 pressure points, 800 nerve endings and 40 odd hair.

11

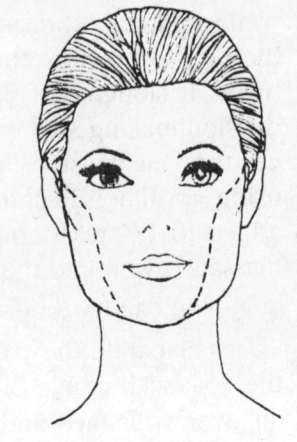

Improving the Skin Complexion and Texture

The skin condition is commonly talked in terms of the complexion and texture. *Complexion* is the visual assessment of our skin colour, tone and clarity. The skin *texture* describes the appeal of our skin to touch. Together, complexion and texture reflect the apparent character and the general health of the skin.

As explained in the previous chapter, different skin types have different complexions and textures. Genes and age are the two unalterable determinants responsible for the differences in the skin type amongst people.

Extreme weather conditions, wrong skin care, use of improper cosmetics and certain skin maladies such as acne and pigmentation also change the skin's colour, tone and texture adversely.

THE "UNALTERABLE" GENETIC AND AGE FACTORS

Let's first understand what is meant by *unalterable* in order to understand the role of the two factors. Genetic factor is an immutable, changeless identity code which we are born with. Age is an irreversible process of nature.

Each individual is different from the others. The differences in the facial features, body structure, skin type, complexion and texture are due to the different genetic codes inherited by the individuals.

Research reveals that people belonging to different races are genetically endowed with different numbers of oil glands, sweat glands, hair and other skin variations. This can logically help us to understand how the skin type, colour and tone differences occur amongst people.

With age, we find that skin loses its qualitative appeal. The skin texture becomes thin, dry and loose. The cell renewal process diminishes with age.

OTHER FACTORS AFFECTING SKIN COMPLEXION AND TEXTURE

The changes in our skin complexion and texture that occur with age are by nature, but the more damaging and serious complexion complications can occur due to wrong nurture. Some of the factors are:

Improper Skin Care

- Improper cleansing of oily skin results in the darkening of the complexion and engenders blemish-causing acne.
- The texture of the oily skin worsens if the enlarged pores are not arrested with proper steaming and toning.
- Moisturizing and nourishing are the most important aspects of dry skin care. If it is not carried out properly,

the texture turns extremely dry and flaky and the complexion looks dull and pallid.

Use of Wrong Cosmetics

- Application of creamy, oil-rich beauty soaps and oil-based chemical make-up products adversely affect the condition of oily skin. The complexion turns sallow yellow and the texture becomes severely thick and greasy.
- Some fairness creams contain mercury drug preparations. They are photosensitive and cause patchy discolouration of the skin in the sun.
- Dry skin treated with medicated or strong soaps loses all its radiance. The texture may feel rough and taut.

Sun

Excessive sun and tan darkens the skin complexion and colour. It can also dry up the skin of its fluid, thereby affecting the finesse of the texture. Certain medications like birth control pills, blood pressure drugs react unfavourably in sun, causing pigmentation or red irritation spots.

Acne

Severe and moderate acne leaves blemishes and temporary dark spots which clear up with time. If the pimples and pustules are picked and squeezed, it causes indentations and small pits on the skin surface. The texture no longer remains smooth.

Apart from acne blemishes, skin irritations, redness and chapping occur in skin disorders of *eczema* and allergies.

Anaemia and Poor Blood Circulation

Dark circles under the eyes, paleness and loss of tone are

common skin irregularities which bother women suffering from anaemia and other circulatory disorders.

CAUSES FOR THE DETERIORATION OF COMPLEXION AND TEXTURE

The most common complexion problem that occurs with time and due to certain other conditions is the darkening of skin colour. The main reason for the darkening of skin colour is the over-absorption of the natural colouring pigment, *melanin*, by the top most cell layer in our skin. Melanin is produced in the basal cell layer and dead cells on the surface absorb this colouring pigment.

A gradual decline in skin rejuvenation and improper sloughing of the skin surface affects the complexion also. The general deterioration in skin is very obvious with age. The diminished blood circulation, the loss in activity of oil and sweat glands and degeneration of body tissue causes dryness and wrinkles on the skin.

CARE OF SKIN COMPLEXION AND TEXTURE

The aspects of skin complexion and texture that need our maximum attention are skin colour, clarity and excessive dryness, roughness and oiliness respectively.

There are a host of potent home-made recipes that can improve our complexion and enhance the texture of our skin.

HOME COSMETIC CARE TO IMPROVE SKIN COMPLEXION

Cleansing Recipe

Instead of soap use gram flour (equal quantities of Green

gram and Bengal gram) mixed in milk or rice water. Scrub the paste on the body and rinse with clear water. This is an excellent recipe to improve the clarity of the skin. Follow this cleansing atleast once or twice a week.

Complexion Masks

- Make a paste of a pinch of turmeric and a tablespoon of milk powder in two tablespoons of honey and the juice of 1/2 lime. Apply it on your face and leave it on till it dries. Rinse your face and feel the difference.
- Take equal quantities of black and white cumin seeds and make into a thick paste with milk or cream. Apply the paste all over the face. After 20 minutes, rinse it off. Use this mask atleast twice a week for maximum effect.

A Simple Lightening Recipe

Take a lime and cut it into two. Rub one half on the face gently. Squeeze the other half in a cup of water, add a little rock salt and drink it. Do it for six to eight weeks regularly day after day and observe the remarkable improvement.

For Blackheads and Acne Blemishes

Make a fine paste of turmeric rhizome and mustard seeds and apply on the spots each night. Wash the spots with water and see them gradually fade away day by day.

HOME-MADE COSMETIC CARE FOR BETTER TEXTURE

Moisturising the Oily Skin

Use an oatmeal and sandalwood scrub (1 teaspoon oatmeal,

1/4 teaspoon sandalwood powder) to cleanse the skin. Follow it with toning with a teaspoon vinegar in a glass of water (Chapter 1). Cut some slices of raw potato and put them all over the face and leave on for 15 minutes. Use the recipe regularly for smooth and moist texture.

Moisturising the Dry Skin

After cleansing the skin with soft soap, tone it with rose water, apply a spoon full of glycerine to which a few drops vitamin oil or *amla* oil have been added on the face. Rinse off after 20 minutes. Use this moisturising preparation on the face for a soft and smooth texture.

Facial for Smooth Texture

Beat an egg in the juice of one lemon and apply this mask on the face and neck. After 30 minutes, rinse it off with clear water. Use this mask atleast once in a week.

A Mask for Chapped Skin Texture

Prepare a mixture of 4 ounces refined linseed oil, 8 ounces rose water, 1/4 ounce of *tincture benzoin*. Mix together and use it every night and morning.

Other Tips

- Yoghurt is ideal to massage skin as it can tone up both dry and oily skin.
- A glass of lime juice has adequate Vitamin C to improve the skin colour.
- White radish and carrot juice taken in plenty provide the essential Vitamin A for smooth skin texture.
- Honey has Vitamin B Complex which is really important for good skin colour. A diet of cucumber, onion, fenugreek improves the complexion.

Hair, Skin and Beauty Care

Warning

To prevent damage to your complexion, you should avoid:

- Perfumed lipstick applied on face in place of blush-on.
- Creams that are highly alkaline.
- Bleaching and lightening creams containing mercury.
- Strong soaps and detergents for cleansing.
- Picking of acne pustules and pimples.

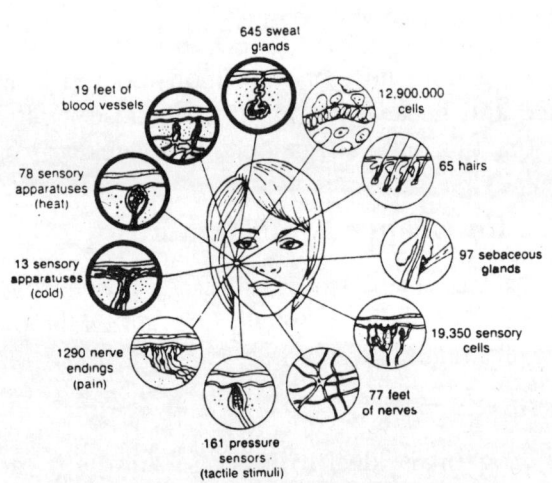

Sensor points of one square inch of skin. Screened area indicates those controlled by pituitary gland

- 645 sweat glands
- 19 feet of blood vessels
- 12,900,000 cells
- 78 sensory apparatuses (heat)
- 65 hairs
- 13 sensory apparatuses (cold)
- 97 sebaceous glands
- 1290 nerve endings (pain)
- 19,350 sensory cells
- 161 pressure sensors (tactile stimuli)
- 77 feet of nerves

MASSES OF BACTERIA

CLOSED COMEDONE

BLACK HEAD

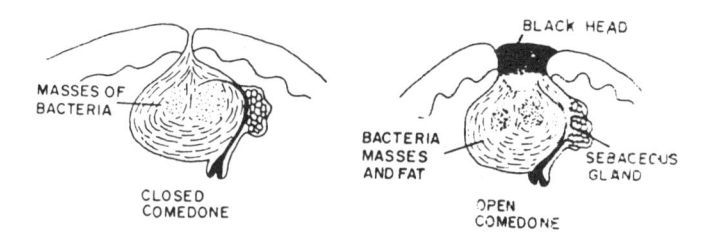

BACTERIA MASSES AND FAT

SEBACEOUS GLAND

OPEN COMEDONE

12

Dealing with Acne

Acne is the most common skin disorder which predictably occurs first during the teenage. It is estimated that over 70 per cent adolescents are affected by a recognisable form of acne.

A lot of research has been done on acne, but there still is no conclusive medical theory as to what really causes it. The visible acne in the form of blackheads and whiteheads is closely associated with hyper activity of the oil glands and congestion of the skin pores.

Seborrhea or excessive oiliness on the skin surface is the general precondition to the formation of acne. However, the what, how and why about seborrhea are not well established.

In reality, there is no treatment that cures acne. The cure lies in the preventive care, the do's and don'ts that have to be followed. With the preventive care, we aim at removing and nullifying the conditions that promote and aggravate acne, and help in building a healthy environment on the skin surface to resist acne.

WHERE IT APPEARS

Acne tends to afflict mostly on the face, back, chest and shoulders.

The reason is the oil glands and the hair follicles, where the acne infection begins, are found in over abundance in these parts of the body.

Usually it is a bad case of severe infection if acne is spread all over. The number of the areas affected is a good measure of the extent of the acne problem.

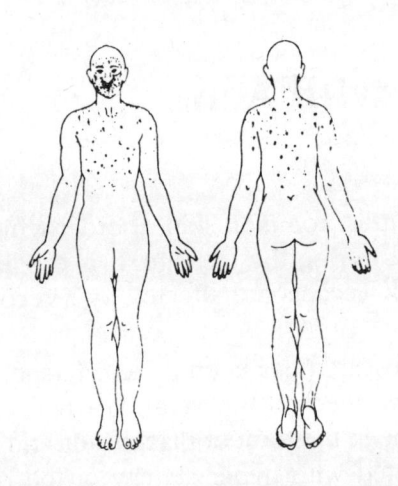

THE MOST COMMON FEATURES OF ACNE

Most people do not have any problem in recognising acne. But sometimes, there are a few other kinds of skin condition that resemble acne closely but are actually quite different.

In order to identify and estimate the acne condition in various stages, there are certain features to be examined.

1. Excessive oiliness on the skin.
2. Whiteheads which sometimes are inflamed spots.

3. Blackheads.
4. Large visible skin pores.
5. Little bumps under the skin (clusters of them).

HORMONES AND THE OILY SKIN CONDITION

The activity of the oil glands is controlled by the male sex hormone *androgen* present in the body. This hormone is present both in men and women in differing proportions.

As and when the level of androgen due to the hyperactivity of adrenal glands and ovaries in the case of women rises, it assumably results in the over-activity of oil glands. This worsens the oily skin condition and encourages the formation of acne.

THE ROLE OF BACTERIA IN THE FORMATION OF ACNE

There are two main types of bacteria and a yeast type of fungus that are all over the skin surface. They are harmless and benign on normal skin. However, they become harmful bacteria on oily skin.

The harmful bacteria work like this—when blockages or congestion appear in the skin pores, the harmful bacteria thrive in the low oxygen environment inside the glands and chemically change the triglycerides into fatty acids. Thereby, it causes the formation of whiteheads.

THE COMMON TYPES OF ACNE

There are basically five types of acne, and they are:

Mild Acne *(Juveenile Acne)*

This is the most common acne condition which affects the teenagers a great deal. So much so that the condition is commonly called *teenage spots*.

The skin examination reveals a lot of little papules and blackheads on a background of greasy skin.

This types of acne does not continue for long without a break. It may last a few months, disappear for some weeks and then start again.

The mild acne conditions is the easiest to treat. Mild acne can potentially turn into a severe form of acne, and the most likely reason for it is usually improper or inadequate skincare.

Scarring in mild acne is not common. Few pits remain after the spots have dried up.

Moderate Acne *(Acne Vulgarias)*

In about 10 per cent cases suffering from mild acne, the condition worsens due to the prolonged existence of acne and severe oily skin condition.

The population and the concentration of whiteheads increase and a large number of papules develop.

The affected spots turn red due to the ruptured blood vessels.

Generally this type of acne improves in the late teens and early twenties. Scarring is minimal and spots clear up after some time.

Severe Acne *(Chronic)*

Only a very small proportion of people enter the state of severe or chronic acne.

The real difference between this and moderate acne is

that the red acne spots are more in number, larger in size, infected and painful to touch.

The entire face, shoulders, back can be affected and infested with the acne spots. It usually takes much longer time to treat this condition and scarring occurs if the spots and pimples are picked.

Picker's Acne

Some young women develop spots that are quite unnoticeable to our naked eye. When examined closely they look different from the usual acne pimples.

The central part of the spot is not like the tip of pimple but is covered by a scab or looks raw. This is because the spot has been picked and scratched frequently.

Even though these spots are not obvious, some women feel very uncomfortable and conscious about them.

Cosmetic and Fringe Acne

This occurs mainly on the forehead and is mostly due to excessive oil and grease, which clogs up the hair follicles.

FACTORS AGGRAVATING ACNE

Continual Touch and Picking

An on-going irritation, pressure applied, picking, wearing tight sweat bands and rubbing increase the acne and heighten the risk of scarring.

Cooking and Frying

Household women cooking heavy and deep fried food are exposed to flying grease or oil particles in the air and fumes. It can worsen their acne condition.

Hot and Humid Weather

Intense heat and humidity often lead to excessive sweating. This coupled with low evaporation of sweat irritates the acne condition.

Vitamin B_{12} Deficiency

A highly inflammatory form of acne is not uncommon amongst anaemic women who require frequent doses of Vitamin B_{12}.

Iodine-rich Foods and Drugs

Spinach, toothpastes, asthma and cold remedies contain iodides, bromides and flourides. Research shows they adversely affect the acne condition.

Hysterectomy and Menopause

In these conditions, the level of estrogen in women drops, resulting in an out of proportion dominance of androgen. Sometimes this results in an outbreak of acne and hairiness.

Use of Wrong Cosmetics

Unfortunately, some of the skin creams, make-up products contain derivates of fatty acids and oils which are potent acne-stimulants. The biggest culprits amongst the skin-care products are the vanishing creams which have high absorption rate.

Prolonged Stress and Anxiety

The acne condition is also worsened by stress. For example, students appearing for examination have to cope with a sudden outbreak of acne.

TREATMENT OF ACNE

There are two aspects of the treatment, the first is the medical drug treatment and the second is the skincare suggested by an experienced cosmetologist.

Medical Treatment

Medical treatment is suggested only in cases of chronic or severe acne and should be taken from the dermatologist.

To outline the drug treatment, it aims chiefly to:

- Cut down the bacteria in the hair follicles and on the skin surface.
- Open the hair follicles by removal of the blackheads.
- Cut down the acne inflammations.

The treatment is rendered by the drugs that can be applied on the acne spots (locally) and those which can be consumed orally.

Local Drug Treatments

The local drug preparations are made of an active chemical compound (drug) and a vehicle or medium compound in which the drug is dissolved.

In recent years, *Benzoyl Peroxide* preparations available as gels and lotions have become very popular in the treatment of acne. Cream "Ultra Clearasil" is a very potent *Benzoyl* preparation. One of the main action points of *Benzoyl Peroxide* is to kill bacteria. It releases oxygen which helps in killing anerobic bacteria.

Usually, one daily application is sufficient, but two may be recommended in case of stubborn acne. The acne condition improves in two to three weeks of continual application.

The *Benzoyl Peroxide* can have one side-effect—it can

excessively dry up the skin. Some women can be allergic to *Benzoyl Peroxide*. Which is why this drug treatment needs a careful administration.

The sulphur drug preparations, available as creams, gels and lotions, are extremely effective in treating acne. Like *Benzoyl Peroxide*, sulphur is committed to killing bacteria. Sulphur is a disinfectant and used in skin treatments for eczema, etc.

In treating acne, sulphur drug preparations work in other ways too. It loosens and dislodges the blackheads from skin pores by causing the skin to peel.

The skin condition begins to improve within two to three weeks. There are no major side-effects. However, it is good to test whether the patient is allergic to sulphur or not.

The Eskamel cream available in the market is a very potent sulphur drug preparation for acne.

Tetracycline usually has no side-effects and hence is the safest drug. However, in some uncommon cases, it causes bilousness, indigestion, vaginal thrush or rash. A precaution: tetracyclines are not recommended during pregnancies.

Note: Keep out of the sun when taking tetracycline—it causes photosensitivity.

The other antibiotics which are prescribed in place of tetracyclines are erythromycin and ampicillin. Another precaution: if you are allergic to penicillin, ampicillin should not be used at all.

DAILY SKIN CARE

Be most conscientious in following your daily skin care routine. There must be no skipping of any step until the condition is corrected.

In the Morning

Wash your hands thoroughly, moisten your face with warm or running water, and wash with a medicated or antiseptic soap (don't use a washcloth—it can shelter the very bacteria that must be stamped out). Choose a light liquid cleanser with ingredients that inhibit the growth of blemish-causing bacteria. Rinse thoroughly with clear running water. Pat dry with a clean soft towel.

Saturate a cotton pad with an astringent, medicated lotion and gently press over the entire face or rinse with cool water to which a few drops of *Tr. Benzoin* have been added. This will freshen, reduce excess oiliness and refine the texture of the skin.

Apply a medicated cream on all pimples. One that is greaseless and skin-tinted will not be obvious on the skin. This will work to dry and heal the pimples. Apply Calamine to which a drop of clove oil and mint oil has been added on all pimples.

Mid-day

Repeat the morning treatment if possible. Otherwise "quick-clean" with the astringent medicated lotion and reapply the medicated cream on blemishes.

Night

Repeat the morning treatment. Sometimes there may be some dry areas such as on the throat, under the eyes, sides of the face. Use an appropriate moisturizing or lubricating preparation. Never apply an emollient cream to any blemished area.

Twice Weekly

Deep-cleanse with a friction-wash to control blackheads and keep the pores free from clogging of excess oil. Wet the face with warm water. Pour about a teaspoonful of cleansing granules into the palm of one hand, add just enough water to work into a creamy foam. Apply to the face with finger tips, concentrate on blackheads and areas of excessive oiliness. Massage gently for a few seconds and rinse thoroughly. Oiliness and blackheads can pose a problem on shoulders and back too. Use the cleansing granules to friction-wash this area when you are in the shower and apply a healing medicated cream to any eruptions before dressing.

The Do's and Dont's

- Avoid using oil-based creams, ointments and make-up products.
- Do not rub, squeeze or pick pustules.
- Follow the skin-care routine scrupulously.
- Do not use any beauty soaps or moisturizers.
- Try to live your life as stress-free as possible.
- Supplement your diet with additional Vitamin B_{12}.
- Avoid deep-frying while cooking as you are exposed to flying grease.
- In case of severe acne, consult a doctor.

MYTHS vs FACTS

There are a lot of misconceptions and myths about acne. While some of these beliefs are unscientific and baseless, the others can be qualified with reliable facts.

Improper Hygiene is a Leading Cause of Acne?

It is both true and false. If proper cleansing is not carried out, it can aggravate the acne condition. However, if the hygiene routine is carried to the extreme with harsh or excess washing and scrubbing, it can ironically worsen the condition.

Long Hair can Aggravate Acne?

The length of the hair cannot be a potential problem at all, as long as the hair is cleansed properly. It is not the length but the improper cleansing of the hair which can aggravate the acne condition.

Acne is more Common among Girls than Boys?

Wrong. It is the other way round. Acne is more common in boys because of the dominance of male hormone androgen.

Acne is Contagious?

False. The trouble-making bacteria are buried deep within the skin and the condition is never contagious.

Masturbation Makes Acne Worse?

This is wrong and is absolutely groundless.

Eating Certain kinds of Food can Cause or Aggravate Acne?

Partly true. Research shows that traditionally forbidden fried food, chocolates, colas and dairy products do not adversely affect the acne condition. Fats which have been eaten, assimilated and circulating in the blood stream have no semblance to the fats within the oil glands. So technically speaking, even the greasiest food is no problem.

However food rich in iodide, such as cabbage, spinach, wheat germs trigger acne-like eruptions.

Eating Certain Food can Help Cure Acne?

There is no definite evidence to prove this.

WARNING WATCH FOR ACNE-CAUSING CHEMICALS

(On your Cosmetic and Make-up Product Labels)
- Isopropyl Isosterate
- Butyl Stereate
- Myristyl Myristate
- Isopropyl Palmitate
- Isocetyl Palmitate
- Decyl Oleate
- Isosteryl Neopentanoate
- Octyl Palmitate
- Octyl Stearate
- Iodoptopyl Lanolate
- Acetol Acetulan
- Amberate P
- Crude coal tar
- Lanosterin
- Laugogene
- Sterolan
- PG 2 Myristyl Propionate
- Acetrylated Lanolin
- Ethylated Lanolin
- D & C red dyes (common in blushers)

HOME-MADE COSMETICS

Cleanser

Apply *Milk of Magnesia* (easily available in the market). Leave on for 10 minutes. Rinse off.

Disencrusting Formula *(Helps blackheads come out easily)*

Dissolve a teaspoon of *Epsom salts (Magnesium Sulphate)* in a cup of hot water. Apply to the acne areas with cotton wool. A papaya-mint tea bag dissolved in a cup of hot water and applied on the acne areas also acts as a discencrusting lotion.

Excellent Toner

Add about 2 to 3 drops of *Tr. of Benzoin* to a mug of cold water. Rinse face with this. It is antibacterial.

Pack

To 2 teaspoons of egg white, add 2 pods of crushed garlic and 1 teaspoon of calamine. Leave on face for 20 minutes, then rinse off.

Moisturizer

A bottle of rose water, 1/4 teaspoon vinegar, 5 drops of glycerine, 2 drops of camphor.

Dryers of Pimples

Touch the pimples with *spirit of camphor*. Keep applying until the pimples dry up. It may "sting" but don't worry. It will check the infection.

To Lighten Scars

Take 1 bunch of green grapes, moisten with water and sprinkle with 1 tablespoon alum and 1 teaspoon salt. Wrap grapes in foil and bake in slow oven for 15 minutes. Squeeze the juice of grapes and cover face with the liquid, rinse off after 15 minutes with lukewarm water.

Use an Ice Pack regularly, wrap ice cubes in a bit of cloth or cotton and apply to the open pore areas. This helps diminish enlarged pores.

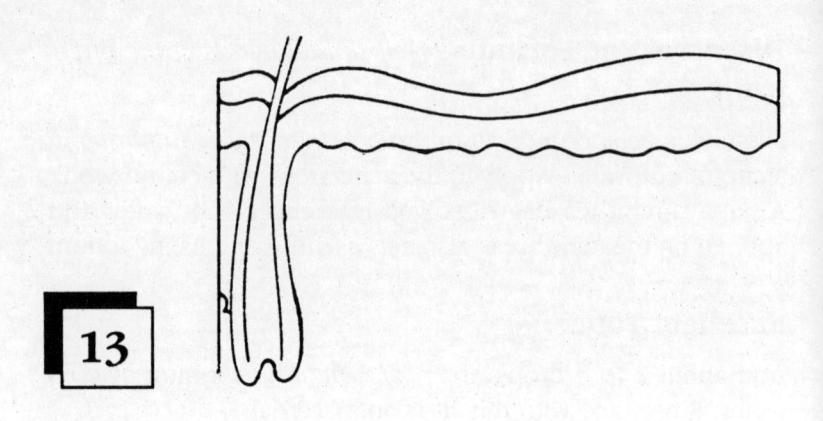

Closing the Open Pores

Our skin has thousands of tiny outlets not visible to the naked eye. These pores carry out the important function of eliminating water, salts, uric acid and oily secretions from our body.

An inadequate elimination of the toxic cellular waste leads to the poor health of the skin, infections and other skin disorders. Many times when our skin pores have to cope with an unusually high and excessive excretion, they enlarge in size giving the skin an unsightly look. The normally not visible pores become visible to our naked eye.

In other cases, when blockages appear in the skin pores, it results in the over-accumulation of the secretions within the glands in our skin. These are finally released by rupturing of the skin leaving gaping pores behind.

HOW THE OPEN SKIN PORES ARE FORMED

The problem of enlarged pores is commonly associated with excessive oiliness and acne. The excessive oiliness of the skin is in turn trigerred by the hormonal changes in the body.

It happens when the male hormones in the body become overly dominant during puberty. The activity of oil glands which is controlled and regulated by the male hormones increases fervently. The skin in order to cope with the over-production of oil secretions has to manage its increased elimination. As the traffic of the oil effusion increases, the mouth of the pore enlarges.

FACTORS FOR THE FORMATION OF ENLARGED PORES

There are three main factors which are directly responsible for the formation of enlarged pores.

Deliberate Picking and Touching of Acne

The worst scarring and pits are a direct result of this. Artificial openings made in the skin to release the effusion from the whiteheads, pustules by squeezing, turn into pits and uneven indentations.

Improper Cleansing

Proper cleansing is foremost in every kind of skin-care routine. Unless the dead skin surface, make-up and grease are removed, they tend to deposit in the skin pores and restrain the flow of oil. The oil deposits attract grime and grease and apply pressure on the mouth of the pores to widen it.

Use of Wrong Cosmetics

Beauty soaps enriched in oil, make-up products that are oil-based, and creams worsen the oily skin condition and therefore their use is prohibited. Acne and enlarged skin pore conditions are aggravated with the use of such cosmetics.

Treatment of Large Pores

Large pores can be easily dealt with proper cleansing and frequent toning of the skin. A large number of vegetables and fruit and herbs help in tightening the enlarged pores. Steaming of the face for five minutes before toning is also helpful. First, follow the cleansing routine as explained in Chapter 10 and then the home-care for arresting the skin pore size as given below.

HOME-MADE COSMETIC CARE

Skin Tightening Mask

Peel a cucumber and whip it up with two egg whites. Add one teaspoon of lemon juice, 2 tablespoons of brandy and half a teaspoon of ground mint optionally. In case the mixture is watery, add some *Kaolin* (white clay) to the extent that the mixture turns thick. Make a generous application of the paste on the areas with large pores and leave it on for 20 minutes. Rinse off with clear water. Use this recipe at least twice a week.

Herb Helper

Buy some *camphor* powder from the chemist. To a tablespoon of *Kaolin*, add a pinch of camphor, a tablespoon of honey and few drops of brandy. Apply it on the face and leave it on for twenty minutes before rinsing it off. Instead of camphor, *alum (phitkari)* powder works equally well. Use the recipe daily.

Tomato Mask

Explained in Chapter 1.

Corn Meal/Oat Meal Mask

Make a thick paste of corn meal or broken wheat (*dhalia*) in some butter milk or cucumber juice. Use it on the face for fifteen minutes and rinse it off. Apart from treating the large pores, this mask helps in improving the texture of the skin.

Large Pore Astringent

Mix one and a half ounce of cucumber juice, one ounce of *Benzoin* available with chemist, about an ounce *Cologne* (perfume) in 5 ounces of rose water. Use this mixture several times during the day to clean the oily skin.

DO'S AND DONT'S

- Do not pick or squeeze acne whiteheads, pustules and papules.
- Apply minimum make-up if the skin condition is extremely oily.
- Cleanse your face atleast three times a day with a light soap and water.
- Use an alcohol-based astringent several times a day to tone the skin pores.
- Use water-based cosmetic and powder make-up product.
- Follow the home-made cosmetic care religiously.

The home-care toning routine is a convenient way of dealing with large pores. It is important to use the astringent especially after the acne, whitehead or blackhead is picked to close the pore.

Apart from the recipes explained, vinegar in water, milk, yogurt, tomato and almond meal are the other food products effective in treating the skin pore condition. They can be used in the form of lotions and facial masks.

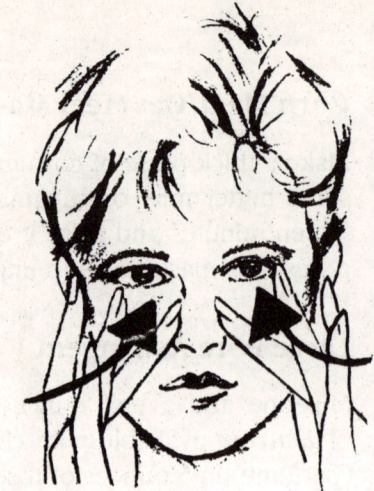

14

Clearing up Pigmentation

Pigmentation is a disorder of skin complexion and colour. It occurs mainly due to the malfunctioning of the endocrine glands and the liver.

The pigmentation problem occurs as either an excessive colouration and darkening of the skin or a loss of colour and pigment in the skin, over the entire body or just in patches and spots.

Pigmentation is more widespread amongst the middle-aged women. Very few women in younger age suffer from pigmentation, and the extent of the problem is minimal with few exceptions. This in fact is related to the endocrinal changes that occur when women reach middle age.

The severity of pigmentation problem is associated with several diseases and disorders. To understand the unusual occurrence of pigmentation, we need to understand these internal disorders.

THE INTERNAL DISORDERS THAT CAUSE PIGMENTATION

Pigmentation of the skin is a symptom common to several

internal disorders. We ought to make a correct diagnosis of these diseases and disorders so as to effectively clear up the pigmentation.

An outbreak of dark freckles and spots all over the body could be due to Addison's disease. This disease causes the damage and impairment of cortical part of the adrenal glands.

Due to over-absorption of iron from the food in the intestinal tract. a bronze pigmentation appears all over the body.

The skin gains a brownish pigmentation or the colours of other compounds also malabsorbed. For example, Women using nasal drops regularly absorb excess quantities of silver present in the drops and develop a silver grey pigmentation in the skin.

Jaundice is another cause—The skin turns yellow due to the presence of excess bile in the blood and the body tissue. This disorder appears when the liver becomes incapacitated or when an obstruction appears in the bile tract.

Sometimes, during pregnancy, dark brown spots appear predominantly on the face. The main reason for these brown spots is the hormonal imbalances caused during the pregnancy.

When the skin turns bluish or purplish, it is due to the lack of oxygen in the blood. The oxygen-poor blood is bluish-red in colour. Women suffering from pneumonia, long diseases and some heart problems are troubled with this type of pigmentation.

Menopause results in decline in the hormonal level which in turn affects the secretion of the colouring pigment in our skin. In case of surgical menopause by removal of ovaries and uterus, the pigmentation is more obvious and severe in nature.

Amoebiasis is a chronic intestinal disorder. It causes excessive purging of the bowels, dehydration and results in sallowness of the complexion and loss of colour.

Deficiency of Iron, Calcium, Vitamin A, E & B Complex results in patchy and spotty discolouration of the skin.

Lack of Vitamin A results in thickening and darkening of the skin. Vitamins E and B Complex deficiency can cause excessive skin pigmentation problem.

HOW IS THE EXCESSIVE PIGMENTATION CAUSED

As explained in the earlier chapter, the production of the colouring agent *melanin* in our skin is influenced by the hormones produced by our endocrinal system. Certain internal conditions such as menopause and disorders have adverse effects on the endocrinal system causing hormonal imbalance. This further results in an over-secretion of the colouring pigment.

Coupled with this, an excessive keratinization, a condition characterised by the presence of the unexfoliated dead cells on the skin's surface causes the darkening of complexion. In fact, our horny skin surface absorbs excessive melanin and therefore appears dark.

In the other condition of liver disorder, it is found that excess bilirubin seeps out of the blood vessels into the spaces between the tissue cells. This imparts a yellow complexion to the skin.

EXTERNAL FACTORS CAUSING PIGMENTATION

There are three external factors that cause pigmentation of the skin.

Excessive Sun

Over-exposure to sun without a shield tans and darkens the skin tone. The ultraviolet rays of the sun penetrate the skin and damage the skin cells also.

Use of Wrong Cosmetics

Certain make-up products which have chemical colours, creams which have mercury drug preparations react adversely on the skin's surface. The result is pigmentation.

Oral Medications

The drugs prescribed for high blood pressure, asthma, diabetes, insomnia and birth control and acne have an unfavourable effect on the skin. More often than not, these drugs cause spot pigmentation.

CLEARING UP THE PIGMENTATION

Bleaching and skin peeling are the two effective methods followed by the cosmetologists to clear up excessive pigmentation. The good thing about these methods is they can be done at home safely and easily.

HOME-MADE COSMETIC CARE

- Bleaching at home—Milk is considered one of the most natural and best bleaching co-agent traditionally. So buy yourself a box of whole milk powder (WMP) preferably or else of skimmed milk powder (SMP) and follow this routine.
- Take two tablespoons of the milk-powder, and (20 Volume) *Hydrogen Peroxide* enough to make a paste. *Hydrogen Peroxide* is usually available at the chemist shop. (20 volume, represents the strength and not the quantity).
- To this paste, add a few drops of glycerine and apply it on the dark spots.

- Leave it on for about 20 minutes and then rinse it off.
- After rinsing, if the skin feels dry and taut, use a generous amount of moisturising lotion.
- Zinc oxide is really effective in lightening the blemishes and highly pigmented spots. Use a zinc cream, available in the market by the name of *zincavet*, regularly on the spots.
- Break Vitamin E capsules and mix in a few drops of castor oil and apply it on the deeply pigmented areas. This recipe is extremely good in treating pigmentation.

SCRUBS AND MASKS FOR SKIN PEELING

(a) Mix 1/2 teaspoon of plain sugar granules in your cleansing cream and work it into the skin by rubbing it gently. Rub all over the face but concentrate on blemished spots. The sugar will be absorbed into the skin. Rinse the face with hot water first, then with warm water, then with cool water and finish with a cold splash. In case of oily skin use the scrub twice a week. For dry skin use it once a week.

(b) Crush some almonds or some cereal (broken wheat) and mix it in two tablespoons of honey. Gently rub the granular paste on the face for few minutes. Rinse off with cool water.

(c) Grate the skin of a papaya and mix 1/2 cup of Fuller's earth, the oil of 2 Vitamin A capsules and mix in the paste. Apply the paste on your face, rinse off after twenty minutes.

(d) Make some carrot pulp and mix in it some Fuller's earth to a thick paste. Crush a Vitamin C tablet for good measure. Apply this mixture for twenty minutes and rinse off. You can use these scrubs and masks at least once a week.

Be sure your skin does not get too dry from these treatments. Moisturise the freckled or pigmented areas after treatment. Pat any of the following home-made lotions on freckled or pigmented skin.

- Butter milk is a gentle bleach.
- Equal parts of malt vinegar cucumber juice and rose water.
- Two tablespoons of grated radish (horse radish) simmered in milk and made into a paste.

DO'S AND DON'TS

- In case of uneven skin tone in patches, supplement Iron and Calcium in your diet with the advice of a doctor.
- If the complexion is pale and dull, supplement Vitamin A in your diet to improve colour.
- In case of a severe pigmentation for a long period of time, consult a physician.
- Have a Vitamin B Complex capsule every day. It is harmless as it is water-soluble and the excess is easily flushed out.
- Do not use cosmetics which have colouring agents. Try to avoid or else use minimal make-up.
- Wear a sun block cream before going out in the sun for the day.
- Avoid using oral birth control drugs and sleeping pills. For asthma and diabetes, use only the prescribed dose and use a sun block when out in the sun.
- Avoid distress and anxiety as much as possible.

LEUKODERMA—THE UNEXPLAINED PIGMENTATION PROBLEM

In some healthy persons, a loss of pigment occurs in certain sharply defined areas of the skin. The affected areas look white in contrast to the surrounding skin. The cause for this problem is not understood and there is no satisfactory treatment.

For loss of pigment, apply mustard oil and a few drops of *Tulsi* juice on the affected area for half an hour. Then rinse off.

Oil of Bergamont is available at essential oil shops or perfume raw material stores. A few drops of it rubbed on the affected area before going out in the sun helps to darken the area.

However, the imperfection of the skin tone is often an outcome of certain nutritional deficiencies or the use of photosentizing cosmetics. The home-made cosmetics given in this chapter use natural food and herbs and therefore assure a complete absence of the preservatives and chemicals that can cause pigmentation, allergies and other skin problems.

15

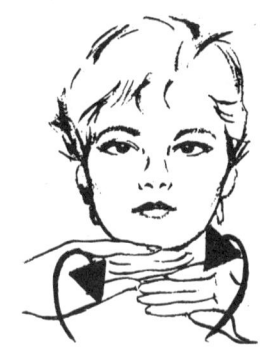

Seasonal Skin Care

Unfortunately, there is never a time of the year when you can relax with your beauty regime. You go through all the trouble in summer to make sure that your skin and hair are thoroughly protected against the sun and heat only to discover that on the return of the colder months, your skin is dry, parched and lacks moisture and you are back where you started.

WINTER

Winter brings its own problems. As the air gets cooler, glands just below the surface of the skin become relatively inactive, so the skin gets drier. Cold winds during winter cause dry red patches alongwith the tight, flaky dry skin.

Even inside your warm cosy home, you could be doing your skin more harm than good by sitting too close to the fire or turning on the heater. The dry air simply drains your complexion of its moisture.

The best way to counteract dryness is to dispense with the use of soap completely. Most soaps are extremely drying to the skin. Use a gentle cleansing lotion or cleansing cream instead. However, if you are a dedicated soap and water lover, then choose a mild soap which has a more moisturising base of glycerine. A good home-cleanser would be the top of the milk blended with a pinch of turmeric powder.

Moisturising is the next important step. Because winter skin usually loses moisture to the environment more quickly than it can replenish it, it has to be protected with extra-rich emollients. These moisturisers help seal in the water below the skin surface and act as a barrier against external conditions. Your routine should include this twice a day, once in the morning and once before you go to bed (after cleansing and toning).

Use a heavier moisturiser than you use during the warm weather months. Apply moisturiser while the skin is damp, evenly over your entire face, massaging cream upward and outwards.

- Every night, before going to bed, take one tablespoon of milk cream and mix in a few drops each of glycerine, castor oil and rose water. Mix well and apply over your entire face, neck and hands. Leave overnight, in the morning rinse with water and splash with cold water.

  This home formula contains oils able to combine with our own to insulate and form a protective barrier on skin cells, keeping moisture in and the harmful effects of the environment out.

  Do not try facial masks and products containing alcohol or lotions as astringents.

- To restore moisture, twice a week, apply a facial mask containing almonds, honey and fats. Leave on for half-an-hour.

- Try this home-made facial mask: 1/4 cup yogurt, 1 teaspoon honey, 1 tablespoon milkpowder, 2 yeast tablets powdered. Leave on for 10 minutes, splash with cool water. Do this once a week for best results.

Use a pot of water over your heater to keep the air in your home moist. Or leave a window open a little to allow some fresh air in.

Do not bathe or wash your face at least half an hour before going out into the cold. Your skin loves water, but water that has moisturised your face will chap the skin when cold air hits it.

Make-up base too can play a part in protecting your face from the cold outside—especially if it is a moisturised foundation. They act, on a smaller scale, in the same way as a moisturiser, but have the added plus of a tinge, of colour to beautify your skin appearance and even out its tone for the perfect complexion. To camouflage uneven colouring and dark circles, try applying a concealer stick under your foundation to be extra sure of a porcelain-like effect.

Slick Lip Tips

Lips have no oil glands of their own, which makes them extremely prone to chapping and cracking in the cold weather. So take extra care to protect them by applying a coat of vaseline overnight and then using lipsalve in the morning. Your salve can be worn either on its own for a subtle sheen or underneath your lipstick.

Don't apply lipstick to chapped lips, it will dry them more. Use moisturiser on your lips several times a day, then apply lip gloss to protect them; or use lip balm with sun screen.

- A home remedy for cracked lips which is very effective: Crush rose petals and mix in a little butter, apply generously on the lips at bed time. This will help keep the lips soft. Touch up your lips with warm creamy colours.

SUMMER (HOT AND DRY)

To combat the dry summer heat, make your own moisturising pack and use twice a week.

- Mash a ripe banana or a watermelon. Mix in 1 teaspoon of milk powder and 1/4 teaspoon of honey. Apply to a clean face and allow it to remain on the face and neck for 20 minutes. Rinse off with cool water.

This pack is especially good for dark skin that gets markedly grey or ashen due to the heat, overwashing and parching winds.

Cultivate an indoor garden. Certain house plants can be skin soothing treatments, filling the environment with moisture and a healthy supply of oxygen. The plants should have wet feet and require plenty of water and be fast growers. The best indoor varieties are *bamboos*, most ferns (especially the *maidenhair* variety), large-leafed plants such as *begonias*, *zebra plant* and *papyrus*.

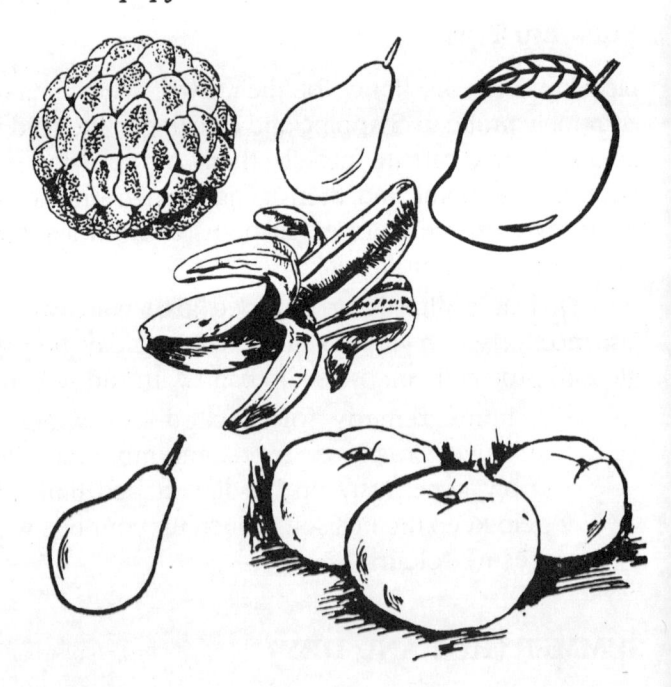

Keep your insides lubricated as well by drinking lots of water.

In summer, even at your oiliest, do not overwash with harsh soaps. Instead, use strong astringents and abrasive pore minimising grains. Try oatmeal and tomato juice pack to shrink large pores and slough off dead skin instead.

- To a tablespoon of tomato juice, mix enough oatmeal to make a thin paste. Add one drop of essential oil of pepper mint.

  Apply to a dampened skin, avoiding the eye and mouth areas. Leave on for 5 to 10 minutes, then wipe off with a damp cotton or a sponge and rinse with cool water.

- To tone down an unwanted shine, add a teaspoon of tablesalt to a spray bottle of water. Mist face with the mixture then carefully rub off with a soft towel.

- Sliced unpeeled cucumber or potato rubbed on the face cuts the shine and is bracing also.

- Before swimming for hours at a stretch in the swimming pool, apply a protective barrier of vaseline to which a few drops of essential oil of lavender has been added.

This protects the skin from the chlorine and preserves the moisture, because the longer the skin is exposed to water, the more the dead cells of the top-most layer absorb moisture and the more they will shrink when they dry out, paving the way for a classic thirsty skin. Lavender prevents burning.

When skin is unprotected, it can burn within a matter of minutes. To protect your skin, you could use a sunscreen which screens out the burning rays or you could use a sunblock to block out the sun completely.

If your skin is especially dry or sensitive, look for products containing P A B A (*Pare-aminobenzoicacied*) and *benzophenones* but no alcohol.

Regardless of your skin type, sunscreens should always be used over moisturiser and under make-up.

- Tea water sprayed on to your face before moisturiser acts as a good home-made sunscreen for a short period out in the sun.

  No sunscreen should give a false sense of security. Even the most potent products still allow a lot of radiation to reach the skin. For a total block, use a sun block like *zinc oxide* or *titanium dioxide*. They are opaque materials that block and scatter light. These ointments are given a flesh colour tint for more aesthetic appeal.

- Apply to sunburned skin every 2 to 4 hours iced water to which a few drops of essential oil of lavender has been added. Iced milk and the juice of cucumber are also very soothing.

- To remove a tan and brighten dull skin, mix one tablespoon oatmeal powdered with enough sour yoghurt to make a paste, and the juice of cucumber or grapes.

  Massage this pack into the tanned areas, leave for 1/2 an hour, rinse off and apply moisturiser.

- Freckles and skin discolourations are aggravated during summer. The powdered root of *manjistha (Indian madder)* mixed into a paste with honey when applied to freckles or skin discolourations will help to lighten them considerably.

SUMMER (HUMID AND HOT)

Cleanse skin often. Three times a week use this exfoliating scrub:

- Mix together *multani mitti* (Fuller's Earth), *Channa Ka atta* (gram Flour) and *Sandalwood powder* in equal quantities. Store in an air tight container. Use a teaspoon of this scrub mixed to a paste with water. This rids the skin of flakes and dirt.

- Use seasonal fruits as facial masks because they are economical and highly moisturising.

  Crush the pulp or squeeze in a blender and apply as quickly as possible before vitamins lose their potency. Grapes are abundant in sugar, vitamins and mineral salts. Use on wrinkles around eyes and mouth. It moisturises, detoxifies and nourishes the skin.

  Papayas are useful on blackheads and blotchy or sallow skin. Cucumber is cooling and improves a dull and greasy complexion.

- Mix the juice of one small cucumber with one teaspoon of rose water.
- Watermelon juice applied to the face and neck freshens up the skin.
- Coconut water rubbed on the skin not only lightens and brightens the skin but also gets rid of heat rash.

  All these lotions should be left on the skin for 15 minutes and then rinsed off with cool water.

  Drink a lot of water to replace the liquid lost through perspiration. It is important to nourish the skin from within.

- Make refreshing eye pads from thick slices of cucumber or cotton pads soaked in milk (iced). To relieve itchy, reddened eyes, use chilled raw potato slices. Place over eyelids and rest for 10 minutes.
- A drop of rose water in each eye at bedtime also brightens the eyes.

Bathing

- Add a cup of buttermilk (*Lassie*) to your bath to tighten pores.

- Nourish and soothe skin with this bath formula. Mix 2 teaspoons salt, 1 1/2 teaspoons almond oil and 1/2 teaspoon malt vinegar and apply to the body before a bath.
- To prevent a tan, apply one hour before your bath, equal quantities of almond oil and malt vinegar.
- To soothe sunburn use a head to toe yoghurt mask. Leave on for 10 minutes, then shower off with cool water. This gives fast relief. Rub ice cubes wrapped in a tissue on pulse points such as wrists and ankles. You will feel instant energy that will wake up your appearance.

Rub the back of your neck and hairline with cologne fresh from the refrigerator.

- To avoid heat rash, remove your sweaty clothes and jump right into the shower. You can relieve the itchiness of heat rash by applying a cooling cornstarch and water. Compress 1/2 cup cornstarch to one pint water.

If you have overexercised yourself or over-exerted and are perspiring a lot, you should drink liquid preparations that contain combinations of water, sugar, salt and potassium which are depleted by the body. *Electral* is a beverage designed for this purpose.

MONSOON (RAINY SEASON)

The rainy season brings along with its share of skin problems—oily skin, open pores, boils, pustules and prickly heat.

If the atmosphere is heavily polluted as in our cities, particles of dirt tend to cling to the skin, giving it a dull grey appearance. Fortunately, frequent cleansing and refreshing will help keep it looking and feeling clean.

- Try this special skin cleaning powder.

Green gram powder—1 tablespoon.

Bengal gram powder—1 tablespoon.
Fenugreek seeds powder—1 teaspoon.
Use a teaspoon of this powder mixed with rose water on your face daily.

- Even if your skin is well balanced or slightly dry, it may be a good idea to change your moisturiser for a very very light weight one formulated for an oily skin which will feel less cloying.
- To combat a greasy skin and open pores—wash your face three times daily with a mild soap. Rinse off every trace of soap with warm water, then cold water. Use an astringent.

Every night, drink a glass of water with a crystal of rock salt and the juice of half a lemon. Use the other half of the lemon in your face mask, mixed with a teaspoon of honey and egg white. Do it everyday for six to eight weeks and see a remarkable improvement in your skin.

During the rainy season, when there is profuse sweating and the body is not exposed to air, red pustules of the size of mustard grains appear on the body, especially chest, back, abdomen and forehead. There is a lot of itching.

- To avoid prickly heat and to soothe it, twice a day dust the body liberally with equal quantities of boric powder, sandalwood powder and talcum powder.
- *Multani mitti* (Fuller's earth) dissolved in water into a thin paste should be applied over the affected parts. When the paste dries, a cold bath should be taken.

Yogurt applied to the affected areas before a bath also helps give relief to prickly heat.

Those of you subject to prickly heat should take cooling drinks and increase the intake of liquids.

Boils are caused by bacterial infection in the roots of the hair. A red swelling forms around the hair and causes a great deal of irritation and scratching. There is pain and sometimes pus.

- To subside the growth in its preliminary stage, apply *kala jeera* (black cumin seed) ground in water over the infected parts.
- For frequent appearance of infected pimples on the face, apply neem tree bark ground in water. The face should also be washed with warm water in which neem leaves have been heated.
- Grated onion mixed with sandalwood powder and applied to the face helps clean septic pustules and makes the skin soft and smooth in a few weeks.

16

Make-up

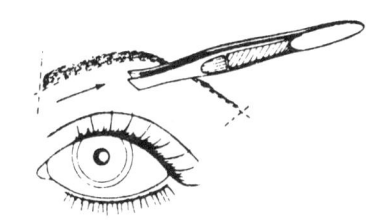

There are three good reasons for applying make-up.

(a) To make yourself prettier naturally. This does not mean

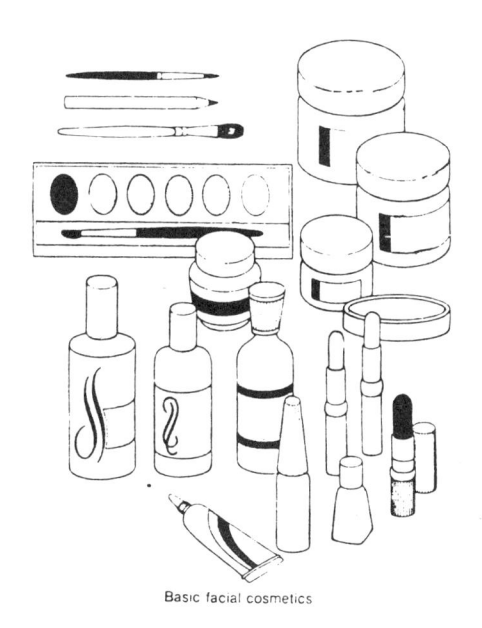

Basic facial cosmetics

you should use a minimum of make-up. Perhaps you should use more than you now use. The trick is to be sure that the shades and texture you choose are ones which make you look as if you just are that lovely, all by yourself.

(b) To highlight your good points and camouflage your bad points.

(c) Make-up protects your skin by acting as an insulator against the elements, if chosen correctly to match the texture of your skin. Now let us proceed with the make-up step by step.

BEFORE APPLYING MAKE-UP

Firstly: Skin should be scrupulously clean. Apply cleansing cream and wipe off with cotton soaked in water.

Secondly: Apply moisturiser on dry skin and astringent on an oily skin. If you have mixed skin, use moisturiser on dry areas and astringent on oily areas. The skin is now ready for make-up.

Foundation: To choose a colour, apply a little on your cheek or inside of your wrist. It should blend in. Apart from that, you should also have a shade darker and a shade lighter.

HOW TO APPLY

Apply light shade to cover dark circles and lines on forehead and nose to mouth lines.

- Apply your foundation. Place a little in your palm and apply it to the face with cotton wool soaked in toning lotion for a more natural look.
- After the foundation has been applied, take a good look at your face. Do you have too round a face, broad nose or a heavy jaw line? You can minimise these defects by using your darker shade.

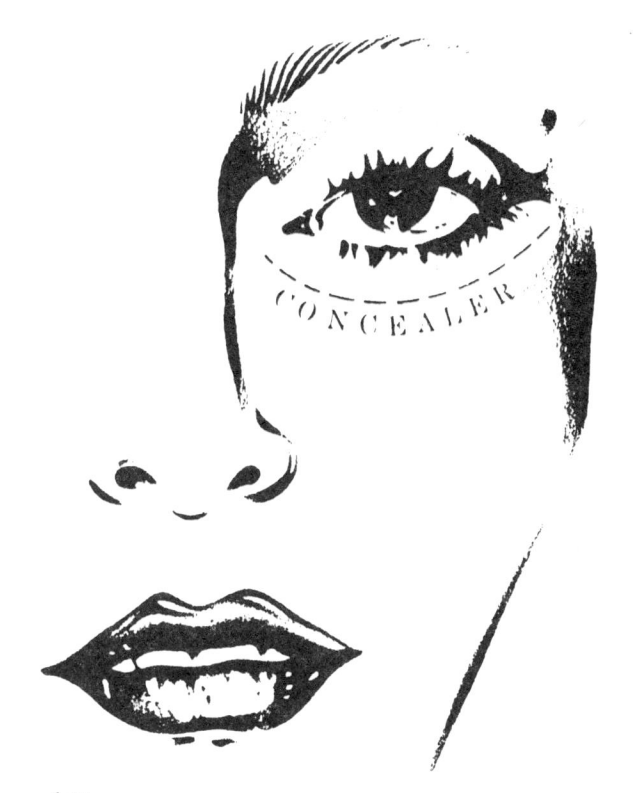

A Round Face
Use darker shade on the sides of the face.

A Large Jaw Line
Apply a darker shade on the jaw line.

A Broad Nose
On both sides of the nose bags under the eyes also can be minimised by using your darker shade under the eyes. Don't forget your neck and ears.

Powder

Translucent powder is the best as it veils and does not cover.

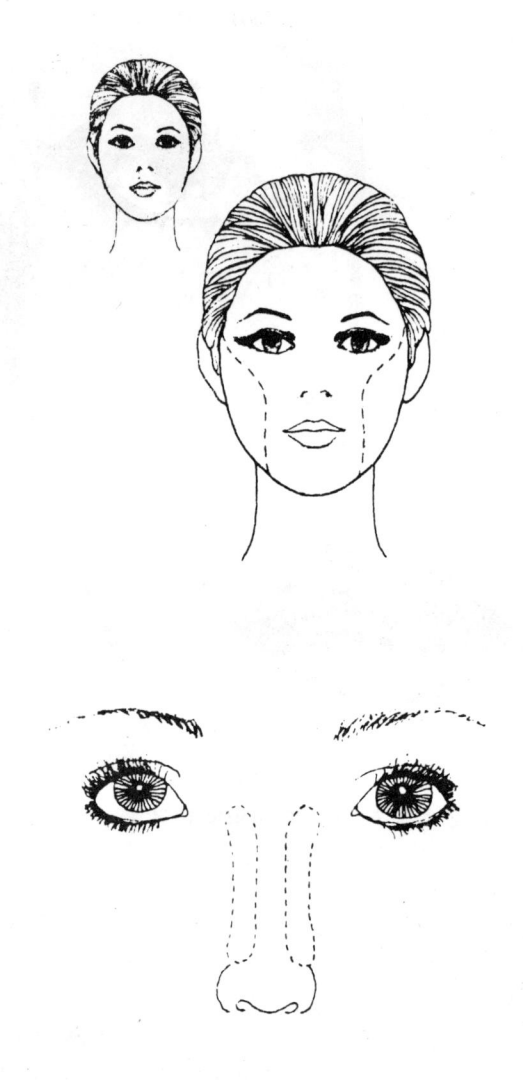

It should only be used if you require a matt finish. Apply with a brush and then dust downwards.

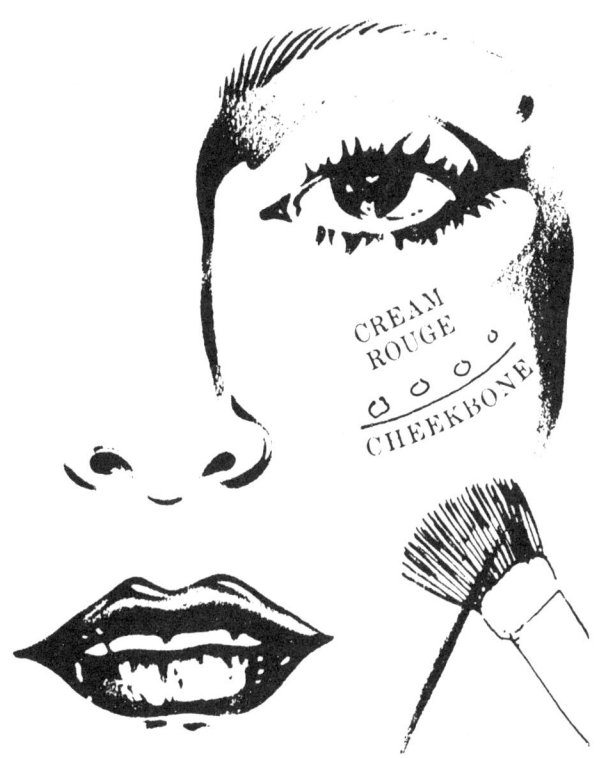

Rouge

Skillfully applied rouge brings a realistic blush to the cheeks. Rouge should be only a whisper of colour.

AGAIN, THE COLOUR YOU CHOOSE MATTERS

Beige or golden complexions should go for colours like tawny, coral or amber

Where to Apply Rouge

It should be placed where your natural blush should be. To find that spot, smile widely with your lips closed, your cheeks

122 Hair, Skin and Beauty Care

naturally rise. Apply rouge on this high area, and fade out gradually towards the hairline.

Note

Never apply rouge too close to the nose and too low on the cheeks. For night time, rouge could be more emphasised because artificial lights tend to rob your face of your glow. Mature ladies could do without rouge or apply a mere whisper of colour if they cannot do without it.

Eye Make-up

Start by having your eyebrows neatly shaped. Get it done professionally for the first time. In case you want to do it at

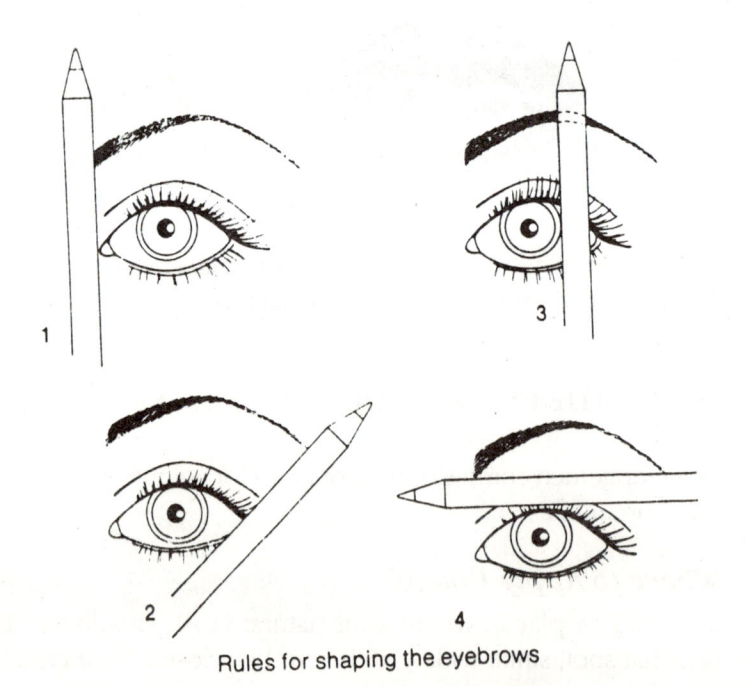

Rules for shaping the eyebrows

home by yourself *never* in between your make-up. The best time to tweeze your eyebrows is after a bath as the pores are open. Apply a little vaseline and smooth into shape. All the hairs that detract from a neat shape should be plucked out. To determine where the eyebrows should start and end, hold a pencil upright from your nose, resting the pencil against the nostril, the pencil should touch the inner edge of the brow. Move the pencil to form an angle ending at the outer corner of the eye. Above where the pencil ends, the eyebrow should end. Tweeze only the stragglers that detract from the clean outline of your brow.

If your face is round or pear-shaped, the outer tips of the brow should point towards the hairline, a long or oval face—the tips should arch down so that the curve will soften the lines of the face.

Eye-shadow

Apply a colourful eye-shadow all over the eyelid area. Don't extend outside the natural shape and don't take it above the eyecrease.

Next, highlight the brow area with white eye-shadow. Contour the eye by applying brown or grey right at the socket line. Next comes the eyeliner, which should be a very thin line drawn close to the lashes. After that comes the mascara which is a must.

Eye-shadow should be skipped by those who have naturally shadowed lids, darkly circled eyes, or wrinkled eye area.

Problem Eyes

Small Eyes, Eyebrows Thin
Pastel or white shadow all over from eyebrow to eyelid and a smudge of brown in the socket.

Prominent Eyes

Deep dramatic eyeshadow to minimise the size of lid. Don't highlight brow, 1/8th inch thick eyeliner extended into inner and outer corners. Make a definite socket line to make the eye more deep set.

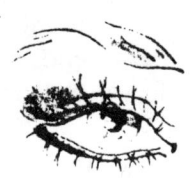

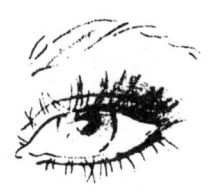

Almond Shape

Pale shadow all over the end and smudge faint brown shadow in the socket. Fine eyeliner all round the eye.

Deep-set Eyes

No socket line. Pastel colours from eyelid and to browbone. No dark shadow.

Lipstick

Lipsticks come in all shades to suit every mood of yours. It is best applied with a lipstick brush. Outline the lips first and then fill in with colour. To make lipstick last, blot lipstick powder lightly, apply lipstick again.

To finish off blot make-up with a cotton pad dipped in icewater and squeezed out.

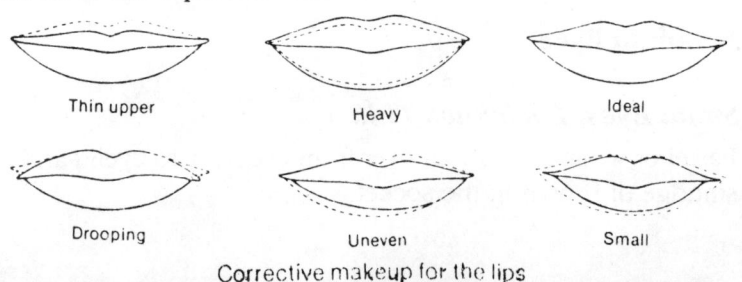

Thin upper   Heavy   Ideal

Drooping   Uneven   Small

Corrective makeup for the lips

THE BODY SECTION

17

The All of you

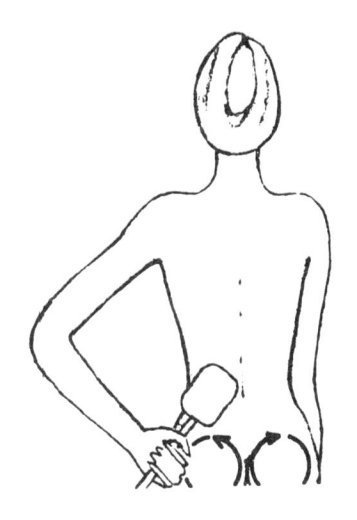

Beauty is the sum of many parts and each should be as perfect as you can make it, if you want to feel attractive, desirable and confident when the glance goes below your neck.

CARING FOR THE BODY

Keeping your body in shape and beautiful is an important part of *Body Care*. First, it heightens your aesthetic appeal, and second, a well-formed body is far more physically competent than a body out of shape. Some parts of our body are vulnerable and deteriorate with age and often lack exercise.

Apart from this, different parts of the body have some typical beauty problems. In this chapter, we focus on how some exercises and beauty routines can help you deal with these common problems.

Neck
It is impossible to see or imagine one's face and figure without including the proportions and condition of the neck. It is like

a rose without a stem. A beautiful, neck, like a good skin is not merely a gift of nature. Very often, the neck which is an extension of facial beauty is neglected and ends up wrinkled and crepe-like.

The neck and the eyes are the areas most highly susceptible to premature ageing. There are various reasons for this and all are easy to counteract provided you keep to a regular neck-care programme. Once the neck has become wrinkled, it is really hard work to rejuvenate it. Your neck responds more slowly to treatments than any other feature apart from the eyes, so be patient and persevering.

Wrinkles appear due to drying of the skin and also due to sluggish metabolism. The main thing to remember is that the supply of blood to this area is particularly lax which results in rough, dull, muddy, or discoloured skin. Exercise combined with massage as well as a regular good skin-care programme and a good posture, is the answer to a beautiful neck.

Extend your regular skin-care regime of cleansing, toning and nourishing to your neck for a flawless complexion. When having a bath, scrub your neck with a rough, soapy washcloth or a dried *thori* scrubber. This makes good sense because scrubbing activates the circulation and removes every trace of deeply embedded grime and dirt. Always clean your neck morning and night with a good cleansing milk and remove make-up with a damp cotton before rinsing. Once a week, use a fine scrub to remove old skin cells and to polish the skin of chin and neck.

- You can make your own scrub by mixing together one tablespoon sandalwood powder and one tablespoon *Multani mitti* (Fuller's earth), as well as enough *Dahi* (Yoghurt) to make a paste. Rinse off after ten minutes.

  Flaky and dehydrated skin responds well to a massage with a good skin food to which a few drops of lemon juice have been added.

- A good skin food for the neck could be made with equal quantities of cold cream, almond oil and rose water. To massage the neck, put a little cream on the fingers of each hand and clasp the base of the neck with the thumbs in front and the fingers meeting behind. Now gently massage from the bottom upwards, until you reach the ears.

To remove dull skin use cleansing and tightening masks. Mix one tablespoon dry oatmeal powder with *Dahi* (yoghurt). Then add the juice of one lime. Massage this pack on the neck and leave for half an hour. Rinse off, pat dry and apply moisturiser. The oatmeal and *Dahi* remove the dead surface cells and the lemon juice restores the acid balance and bleaches the skin. Follow with an almond oil massage.

Back

Be conscious of the way you hold yourself and practice pulling your shoulders back, stretching the spine and not slouching. Do arm swinging exercises, swinging backwards. If you have a greasy skin, the areas between your shoulder blades can get very greasy. Wear cotton instead of synthetic fabrics next to the skin.

- Tackle spots and oiliness with this exfoliative creamy back-wash. Mix half teaspoon salt with a tablespoon of *milk of magnesia* (available at the chemist). Massage into skin and rinse off.

Beautiful Breasts

Female breasts consist of milk glands, lymph ducts and fatty and fibrous tissue. Size is often a matter of fat and glands.

Many women feel their breasts are the wrong shape, lack bounce, are too long/large or too small. A small bust has every advantage. It does not have such a fight with gravity and can stay in good shape for a lifetime. Women with large busts have to take care to support them and to keep them looking shapely and firm.

Women with very large bosoms attempt to hide them by stooping with rounded shoulders which does nothing for the body shape in general. It only encourages the breasts to droop. Whatever size your breasts are, good posture is a must.

- Try this exercise to improve posture. Stand in your usual position. Now lift the shoulders a fraction, move them back about two inches and drop them from this point, so that the back and shoulder muscles lift the pectorals and in turn, the breasts, extending the areas from navel to diaphragm which improves the bust line.

However out of condition your breasts are, they can always be improved with exercise. The most efficient bust conditioning sport is swimming. The breast stroke is best, as the name would suggest.... swim with the head raised out of water and breathe regularly and deeply.

Exercises to improve your bust can be done at any odd moments during the day. Here are three exercises for lifting your breasts.

- Sit cross legged or on your heels like in *Vajra asan* and extend arms behind you, interlacing the fingers, hold the position for a count of 10 and then relax—Repeat three to four times.
- Sit on the floor or a chair and lift arms over head and press palms of the hands together. Using your muscles and still pressing your palms against each other, lower them slowly to shoulder level, count 10—Relax and repeat.
- Clasp hands and push hard against each palm—Repeat whenever you have a spare moment.

Many women wear the wrong size bra which is not good because proper support is necessary. Here is a sizing guide—measure your circumference directly under the bust and add five inches, that is your bra size. If a second measurement around the fullest part of your bust is exactly the same as the bra size, you need an A cup; if it's 1 inch more B; if 2 inches more C, and 3 inch more D.

A bra that is too tight for your back can cause pressure marks under the arms and mid-back: too tight straps leave ridges on the shoulders, ill-fitting cups can accelerate *mastitis* (inflamation of the breasts).

Last but not least, an unused, uncared for body withers and dries up. A 50-year-old woman who is full of sexuality and leads a vibrant life is still making the same tissue forming secretions she did at 30. Women and girls who are depressed, run down or are (or feel they are) unloved, have breasts that are cold to the touch and lack a healthy bouncy quality.

Waist and Tummy

Over-weight and lack of exercise are two reasons why your waist is not shapely. Waists are whittled with exercises and these two exercises are a sure bet.

- Stand with feet apart. Lift arms over head and clasp the head. Bend from the waist towards the left and bounce four times to the right. Repeat six time a side every day.
- To get rid of your tummy bulge lie on your back on the floor with your feet locked under a bed or a chest and cross your hands over your chest. Now bring yourself up almost into a sitting position (it is the almost sitting up that makes you feel the pull.) Then almost go back down to the floor. Do this exercise six times twice a day, if you are keen to banish the flab quickly.

Stretch marks happen when the skin cannot stretch to accommodate quick growth in puberty or **pregnancy**.

Prevention is the answer. If you are pregnant, try lubricating your tummy with a Vitamin E-rich cream or oil and do not let your skin get dry.

To make them less obvious, apply a touch of waterproof make-up with a damp cotton in a colour to match your skin tone.

Legs

Thighs get the flabbiest. Massage them while having a bath and soaping yourself by twisting and pummelling the flesh, to improve circulation. Afterwards pat dry and apply lots of soothing body lotion.

Knees whether they are squashy or knobbly, mostly depends on heredity and weight. If the skin on the body gets dark and dry, use lots of cream. Once a week, massage them with one tablespoon oil (any oil), juice of half a lemon and half a teaspoon salt—before a bath.

Legs tend to be dry-skinned because they don't have very active oil glands, so lubrication with body lotion or cream after every bath is a good idea. Spider veins, which are often round the knees and on the thighs may look unattractive, they could be treated by your doctor with an injection. Varicose veins should not be neglected and need medical treatment, usually surgery. It helps to rest as often as possible with your legs raised.

Shape up with daily exercises for better-looking limbs.

- Stand about two feet away from a support and stretch and lift leg (keeping leg straight), swing across body. Do 20 times. Repeat 20 times with the other leg.
- Stand with one hand resting on a support and kick leg forward and backward as far as it will go. Do 20 times. Repeat 20 times with the other leg.

Hips and Bottom

Heavy hips and a flabby bottom seem to be the problem of many women.

Unfortunately, hip and thigh problems don't normally respond to diet alone. Exercise is really the only way to attain a smooth, firm, proportioned figure.

If you follow the hip and bottom programme outlined here, you will see visible results in two month's time, likely even sooner. Do the following exercises daily. These are super spot-reducers.

- One exercise you can do anywhere is to contract the buttock muscles hard and hold for the count of six.

    If the flab is lumpy and has a dimpled look, it could be cellulite. The problem can be tackled by scrubbing with a *loofah* while having a bath to boost circulation.
- Walk on your hips from one end of the room to the other and back again. Do this daily to slim your hips. Raise right hip, push right leg forward. Now raise left hip, push left leg forward.
- Begin on hands and knees. Draw left knee to chest. Kick left leg back and up, lifting head. Lower leg, draw knee to chest again. Kick rhythmically ten times. Repeat to right.

Apart from these exercises, take up an activity that you enjoy doing, like dancing, jogging, walking, swimming, tennis or cycling. Regular physical activity performed at a fairly strenuous level will slim heavy hips, in addition to promoting all round fitness.

Besides these exercises and a sensible diet, devote at least five to seven minutes a day to massaging the affected tissues.

- Now starting with the flesh on the bottom and working upwards along the hip, pick up the surplus tissue and

gently *knead* it as you would dough, using the knuckles.
- *Wring* the flesh into S bands, using your right hand to guide the tissues in one direction, your left hand reversing the direction. Keep alternating the hand and work as usual from bottom to waist.

Use a creamy body lotion or vegetable oil for your massage as massage strokes are easier with lubrication on this dry area of the body.

Follow this hip and bottom plan for a month. Your tape measure will record measurement changes after 30 days, perhaps sooner.

Apart from the tips given in the chapter, the beauty problems of hands and feet have been discussed extensively in a separate chapter. Cellulite, which is a common problem amongst women is discussed in the next chapter.

Don't just read this chapter but practise it as suggested and feel the difference.

18

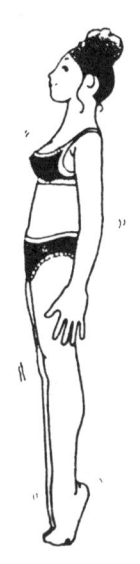

Treating the Cellulite

Cellulite is not a medical term. It is a word coined by the Europeans to describe a common physical condition characterised by the uneven bulges that appear visibly prominent on our body.

The tendency to develop cellulite is largely hereditary. It afflicts young and old, men and women alike.

WHAT IS CELLULITE ?

Cellulite is a combination of excess fat, water and extra-cellular waste which gets lodged in the connective tissues of our body. Once the cellulite is trapped, it pushes up against the network of skin's restraining fibres. It appears as the unsightly unevenly distributed lumps and pads of fat on our body.

Cellulite is different from the ordinary layer of fat which lies beneath our skin. Unlike cellulite, the evenly distributed fat layer provides insulation and cushioning to the internal organs and is a source of energy, our body ordinarily calls upon.

WHERE DOES CELLULITE APPEAR ?

Women are more likely to have cellulite in the prominent areas of their bodies. They have excess fat deposits on their breast and hips while in men, excessive fat deposits are found more often on the abdomen and the upper back, around the shoulders and neck.

WHAT CAUSES CELLULITE ?

Most cosmetologists agree poor diet, poor physical maintenance, internal stress and inadequate elimination are the primary causes of cellulite formation. Food poisoning also causes cellulite.

(a) If our diet lacks adequate calories and nutrients or the food taken is hot and spicy, it results in irritation and aggravation of the digestive and intestinal tract. This produces a stress within our body. This can further be worsened by poor elimination.

(b) Sedentary work life and lack of physical exercise leads to improper elimination and excess retention of the toxic cellular waste (lactic acid) in our muscles. This promotes the build-up of new cellulite.

(c) Excess sodium consumed as common salt leads to the retention of water and a bloated feeling. As a result, it encourages the formation of cellulite.

CONTROL OF CELLULITE

Diet

Dieting to control cellulite formation means eating sensibly so as to avoid stress and help the body cleanse itself of all irritating and polluting agents through the process of elimination.

Diet should consist of four basic food groups—milk, food, meat (fish, chicken), vegetables, fruits and cereals. A well-balanced and nutritious diet is very efficacious in treating cellulite. Consulting a good dietician will help in deciding the correct menu for oneself.

Foods to be avoided are: Spiced meats, highly fatty foods, fried snacks like potato chips, white bread, pastries, excessively salted food, nuts, alcohol and coffee.

Physical Exercises

Besides a balanced diet, one should have a regular and planned exercise programme. It helps the body to dissolve existing cellulite deposits and prevent the formation of new ones.

Regular exercises promote a sense of well-being as well as reduce stress and strains of everyday life. They help in eliminating waste materials within the body which will otherwise contribute to the lumpy fat.

Brisk walking, jogging and swimming promote the healthy development and even distribution of the flesh in the body. If you do not have time for exercise, walking to and from the place of work may help. The busy executive and sedentary workers should find time to relax and undertake at least half to one hour of walking and spot reducing exercises. A word of caution. One should not work into exhaustion which may be counter-productive.

Autolysis

Autolysis means the process of self-cleaning and self-washing of wastes. Periodically, the body becomes steeped with an accumulation of refuse, sludge, impurities, toxic wastes, debris and mucus. Autolysis is a natural way to get rid of the wastes.

Morning Self-washing Fruit Cocktail

The fruit cocktail is prepared as under:

- A cup of sun-dried apricots soaked in pineapple juice overnight is taken first thing in the morning. This cocktail, through the action of the pineapple juice, releases the iron and copper of the apricot which, in turn enriches the blood with life-giving oxygen which is required to awaken and revitalise the circulatory system and create a natural self-cleansing.

Cellular Washing Exercises

Tired and fatigued persons do experience regeneration through natural foods. But in order to free the cement-like sludge and clogged cellular wastes that fester in the intricate circulatory channels, a set of eight simple massage exercises has been devised. These exercises help to loosen up wastes, remove blockage, free eliminative channels and help cast off choking sediments.

1. Use a large bath towel for all exercises. Loop the towel behind the neck. Pull your chin in full forward on both ends of the towel and resist the towel with the neck, as hard as you can, for just six seconds. Do it only once.
2. Now slide the towel down to the small of your back. While pulling forward on the towel, resist by contracting the muscles in your buttocks and your belly. Push back hard against the towel and count to six.
3. Loop the towel under your left foot and pull up with both hands while your foot pushes down.
4. Do the same exercise under the right foot.
5. Now under both feet, pull up with hands, while your feet push down.
6. Take the towel by the far end, hold towel at thighs and pull hard on both ends of the towel.

Treating the Cellulite **139**

7. Now raise the towel high overhead and pull towel hard for six seconds.
8. Now hold towel at shoulder height straight in front of you and pull towel as hard as possible for six seconds.

Stiff Bath Brush Awakens Sluggish Circulation

While taking bath, after soaping, scrub with a stiff bath brush vigorously all over the body. This enhances the blood circulation below the skin which in turn helps to cast off the stored-up fatigue causing lactic acids, carbon dioxide and other chemical abrasives.

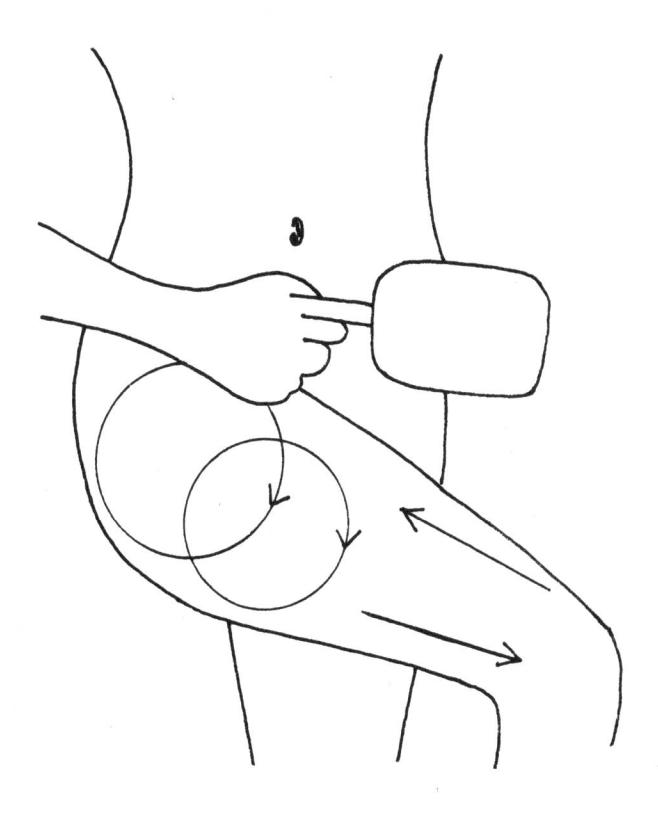

Controlled Juice Fasting

The controlled fasting is an ancient system for washing and resting the internal organs. Most people prefer a day of raw fruit juice fasting. Some like raw vegetable juice fasting. The power of vitamins, minerals, enzymes, amino acids and other valuable detoxifying elements in the juices are able to work without the interference of solid food. Fast only one day per week.

    A regular (night is preferable) tub bath in comfortably warm water helps steam out the accumulated toxins through the pores in the skin.

Home-made Cosmetics

Cleansing Bath: 2 handfuls of *Epsom salt (Magnesium Sulphate)* from the chemist in a tub of hot water. Soak it for 20 minutes.

Massage Oil: Boil Ivy leaves (a handful) and a handful of *Kamal* (lotus) leaves in about 1 litre of sesame oil for 20 minutes. Use the oil for massaging the cellulite areas daily and watch it disappear.

CONCLUSION

The key to success in your battle against the ugly ravages of cellulite lies in just one word **caring**. Caring means to follow meticulously the directions given on diet and regular exercises.

19

Hands

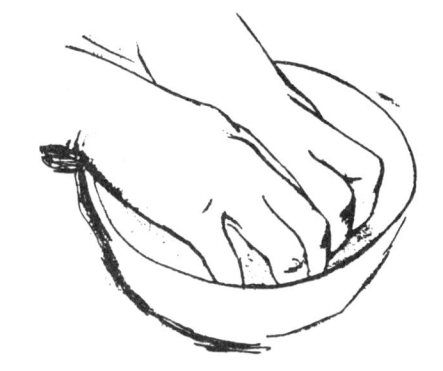

Let's face it, there are some things you just cannot hide and your hands are a splendid example. Like your face, voice and eyes, your hands also express the essential you. They are your ambassadors to the world. So it always seems a pity, if they are neglected, as they let down your whole appearance. Nails talk and speak volumes about how much you care about looking good.

Hard water, detergents, chemicals as well as skimping on hand-drying can quickly lead to rough, sand paper-dry skin. If you persist in using your nails and finger tips to rip open parcels and boxes as well as pretending they're tools to be used for jabbing lift buttons or dialing telephone numbers, you will soon want to hide your hands completely. So, if you've fallen by the wayside, read on, help is here.

One golden rule to follow for good-looking hands is to apply a good, lubricating handcream always after washing. Protection is the secret. Creams and oils do not soften the hand skin, they merely hold in the moisture in the skin and prevent its escape. Hand skin is just as vital to your look as super nails. For harsh chemicals and cold dry air, the answer is protective gloves. For sunlight and sports enthusiasts a sunscreen on their hands that contains Para-Aminobenzoic acid to screen out the aging ultraviolet rays. For biting winds and long exposure to water, petroleum jelly is an inexpensive and effective barrier.

COMMON HAND PROBLEMS

Sweaty Hands

Sweaty hands is the result of a sudden release of 'Cold Sweat' from the eccrine sweat glands of your palms. This is usually a nervous condition, and the only remedy for this complaint is to carry a bottle of eau-cle-cologne in your hand bag, so you can dab a few drops on your palms when needed. Also step up your intake of Vitamin B Complex.

Red Hands and Chilblains

For hands in a constant state of redness and those of you who suffer from chilblains during winter, try this exercise to improve circulation as your whole problem is due to poor circulation.

- Stretch your hands out in front of you and stretch your fingers as far apart as you can, keeping them tense; hold this position for the count of ten and then slowly reduce the tension in your fingers. Repeat ten times daily.
- Shake your hands vigorously several times a day. Apart from this, take a course of *calcium* tablets, and massage your hands daily.

Roughened or Chapped Hands

Roughened or chapped hands are usually caused by a lack of Vitamin B Complex. So take a course of tablets or injections.

Try a compress of an infusion of *Marigold* petals for chapped or roughened hands.

NAILS

Nails are easier to understand when they are compared to hair. Both are primarily composed of dead tissue protein. Nails are healthy when you feel fit and eat a well-balanced diet. Vitamins A and B Complex, plenty of liver, citrus fruits, milk, honey, celery, cauliflower, nuts and grapes are good for the nails. Vitamin D capsules are also particularly beneficial.

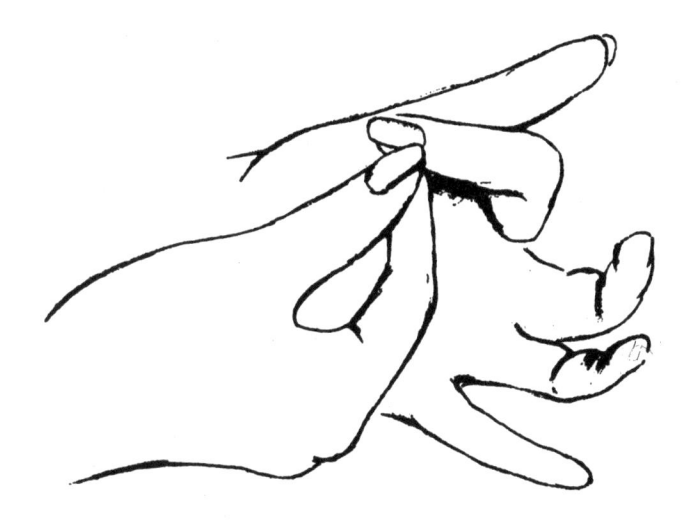

Brittle and splitting nails are caused by lack of calcium. It can be improved by taking two tablespoons of gelatin daily in a glass of fruit juice. You will see the results after six weeks. Ragged cuticles are caused by lack of lubrication. So lubricate with lots of cream, the cuticles and the areas around the nails as often as possible to eliminate raggedness and hang nails.

Nail-biting is often a sign of tension. It is also insanitary. Self-discipline is the only solution to the problem of nail-biting. Also take life more calmly, and keep your nails carefully manicured. When nails begin growing, they may require strengthening. Use a colourless nail hardener.

Manicure

A manicure once a fortnight is very essential for an elegant look. Before every manicure; soak your hands in a little warm olive oil for about 5 minutes.

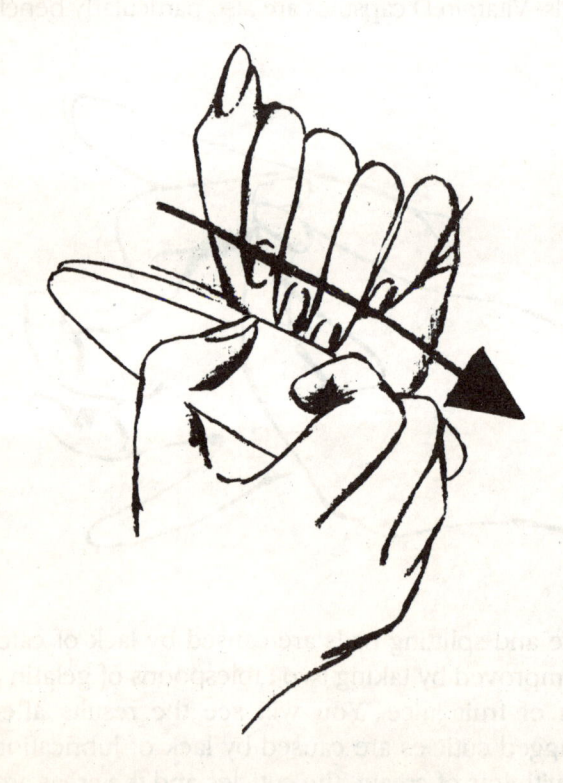

- Shape nails either oval, round or square using the smoother side of an emery board.
- If cuticles are neglected, they tend to stick to the nail.

A healthy cuticle should be soft, supple and not stuck to the nail. Smooth some cuticle cream into the cuticles and push back the cuticles.

- Follow this by removing all the dead cuticle with an orange stick wrapped in cotton and dipped in cuticle remover.
- Snip off hang nails if any with a cuticle cutter but do not cut the cuticle as it would only make the cuticle rougher and harder.
- Massage hands with a good hand-cream.
- Remove all residue from the nails by washing and drying the finger tips.
- You can make your individual hand lotion from the following:

    1/2 cup rose water
    1/4 cup after-shave
    1/4 cup glycerine
    1/4 tablespoon white vinegar

    Mix all together and bottle for use.

- Apply nail polish.

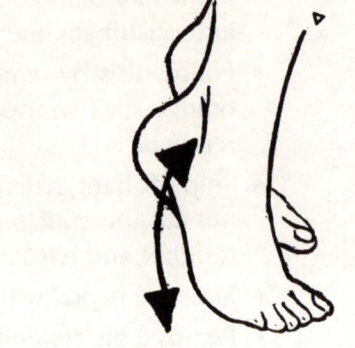

Your Pedestals—the Feet

- The feet are the pedestals of beauty. Your posture, your figure, your grace of movement all depend, finally on your feet. And the expression on your face depends upon your feet. You must have seen the look of strain and misery of women whose feet hurt.
- The human foot has 52 bones, and 214 ligaments. It is subject to more pressure and more injury than any other part of the body. It can also be affected by a great variety of diseases, circulatory disorders, dermatities, diabetes and arthritis.
- However, minor foot problems start from outside pressure and everyday complaints like corns, calluses and ingrowing toe-nails are very painful and could grow worse unless they get proper treatment and attention.

FEET PROBLEMS

Corns and Calluses

Corns and calluses are caused by the way we walk and by

friction on the foot. You are, therefore, better off walking bare foot or with a minimum sandal whenever possible. A massage with olive oil, castor oil or coconut oil softens the dead tissues and makes it easier to rid yourself of these problems.

- A salt foot-bath followed by a massage with lemon peel oil is very soothing. You can make this by turning half a lemon inside out and filling with olive oil or any other vegetable oil. Allow the oil to steep overnight.
- To ease the pain of corns, tape garlic or onion on the corn.
- Rubbing a pumice stone over calluses softened by bathing keeps calluses small and eventually eliminates them.

For Cracked Heels

100 gm coconut oil, 5 gm camphor, 20 gm paraffin wax. Melt and store in a tin. Use on clean feet at night daily till the cracks disappear. Wash feet in the morning and use a hand and body cream.

Itching Feet

Lemon juice and vinegar applied to the feet are excellent for controlling itching feet. Athlete's foot is a fungus which develops an itchy rash between the toes with minute blisters splitting the skin. Onion juice between the toes relieves itching and athlete's foot.

Swollen Feet

Do not be frightened because it is not dangerous even though painful. The swelling will soon disappear—apply hot and cold compresses to the feet.

- Lie or sit with your legs elevated.
- Soak feet in a basin of hot water to which a handful of *Epsom salts* (*Magnesium Sulphate*) and a handfull of salt has been added.
- The swelling will soon disappear if you tie crushed leaves of *geranium* over the feet.

In-Growing Toe-Nails

Are mostly self-inflicted by incorrect trimming of the nail—cutting too short or when snipping down the sides, tearing the nail, resulting in a sharp piece piercing the skin. To heal the wound, new skin is formed and builds up. You should see a chiropodist at the first signs for, in severe cases, the whole nail may have to be removed.

How to Avoid In-Growing Toe-Nails ?

Always cut toe-nails straight across and don't cut corners back into the groove.

Perspiration of the Feet

It should never be suppressed because severe and incurable diseases will follow and will last until the feet perspire again. Use a foot powder.

Make Your Own Foot Powder

Talcum Powder — $1\frac{1}{2}$ cup
Boric Acid — 2 tablespoons
Corn Starch — $\frac{1}{2}$ cup

Mix all the ingredients together and use.

Chilblains

Is due to poor circulation and they react with the cold, damp weather. Scratching an itchy chilblain only makes a broken

Figuring out the Diet

Name	Quantity	Calories
Chicken	1 cup	220
Mutton chop	1	100
Tandoori chicken	2 pcs	450
Fish fingers	3 pcs	162
Sheekh Kabab	2 pcs	300
MISCELLANEOUS		
Tuna	1.5 cup	175
Tuna canned in oil	1.5 cup	170
Sardines canned	1.5 cup	175
Salmon canned	1.5 cup	120
Fish sticks	3 to	150
Crab	2 cups	67
Oyster fresh	1 doz	160
Shrimp canned	1.5 cup	100
Shrimp rolled & fried	1.5 cup	19
Jam	1 tbsp	100
Marmalade	1 tbsp	100
Mayonnaise	1 tbsp	110
Butter	1 tbsp	120
Vegetable oil	1 tbsp	130
Salad oil	1 tbsp	125
Ghee	1 tbsp	140
Sugar	1 tbsp	60
Honey	1 tbsp	30
Horlicks	2 tbsp	41
Ovaltin Bournvita	3 tbsp	38
Papad 1 grilled	1	25
Papad fried	1	43
Mango pickles	1 pc	65
Bhel Puri	One cup	280
Papri	1 plate	25
Pani puri	1 plate	125

Name	Quantity	Calories
MILK & MILK PRODUCTS		
Milk	1 cup	100
Condensed milk	1 cup	320
Skimmed milk	1 cup	45
Butter milk skimmed	1 glass	60
Curds	1 cup	60
Khoa	$1/2$ cup	206
Ice cream	1 scoop	114
Shredded cheese	$1/2$ cup	150
Blue cheese	$1/2$ cup	100
Cheese	$1/2$ cup	82
Cottage cheese	1 tsp	16

MEASURES

Spoon: 2.5" Long diameter Cup: 3 1/4" diameter top
   1.5" short diameter   2 1/2" diameter depth
   0.3" depth   2" diameter bottom

Here's an example of how to figure out a week's diet.

Day 1

Breakfast: Cereal with yoghurt, honey and fruit, tea, fruit juice.

 Main meal: 3/4 cup *paneer* (cottage cheese), baked jacket potatoes, mixed salad dressed with olive oil and lemon juice, fresh fruit salad, one glass of lemon juice.

 Other Meal: Vegetable soup and *phulka*, or slice Brown Bread, glass of fruit juice or vegetable juice, one apple or an orange.

Day 2

Breakfast: Soft boiled egg, whole meal toast, tea and fruit juice.

 Main Meal: Brown rice with tomato and vegetable sauce sprinkled with very little grated cheese, green salad dressed as on day 1. Stewed apple sweetened with honey, if required a glass of lemon juice.

Other Meal: *Palak paneer*, (Cottage cheese with spinach) *phulka*, apple or pear, butter-milk or fruit juice.

Day 3

Breakfast: Oatmeal porridge made with water and served with honey and skimmed milk, fruit juice, tea or herb tea.

Main Meal: Omelette filled with cottage cheese (*Paneer*) and herbs, fresh whole meal bread (lightly buttered) or *phulka*, green salad dressed as before.

Soaked dried apricots sweetened with honey and served with yoghurt (*dahi*), lemon tea or juice.

Other Meal: Sandwich of cold chicken with salad, or cream cheese and salad on wholemeal bread. One apple, orange or pear, glass of skimmed milk.

Day 4

Breakfast: Cereal with skimmed milk, whole meal toast and honey, fruit juice and herb tea.

Main Meal: Stir mixed vegetables (onions, carrots, brinjal red and green peppers, cauliflower and mushrooms cut into small pieces and quickly fried in sunflower or olive oil with yoghurt, lemon tea or lemon juice.

Other Meal: 3/4 cup cottage cheese, tomatoes sliced, lightly buttered whole meal bread, fruit juice or tea or herb tea.

Day 5

Breakfast: Yoghurt with sliced banana and sprinkled with honey, fruit juice, tea.

Main Meal: Grilled lamb chop (or nut and lentil cutlet) with steamed fresh vegetables and salad of raw cabbage, walnuts, apples, carrot, and peppers dressed with oil and orange juice. Stewed plums with honey, lemon, tea or juice.

Other Meal: *Phulka*, or slice of brown bread, 3/4 cup *dal*, 2 glass of fruit juice, one apple or orange.

24

Exercises

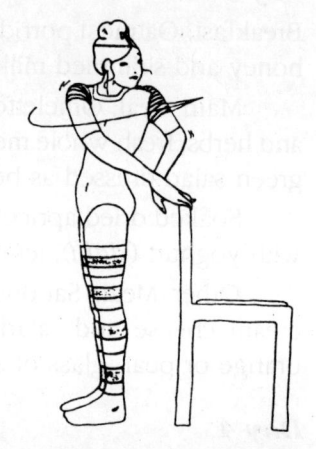

It is virtually impossible to overestimate the value of exercise. It not only gets rid of unsightly flab by toning and firming your muscles, but it is also the world's best tranquillizer, doing away with sleeping pills and helps work off a bad mood and temper. Most cardiologists agree that if a woman exercises vigorously for half an hour, three times a week or more, it helps prevent heart trouble. This is why it is so important that an exercise programme is started the moment you reach 40, if you have not already started one.

As women enter the pre-menopausal and menopausal years, they lose much of their hormonal protection against heart attacks. Exercise keeps blood vessels elastic and builds up circulation. Doctors in America, Europe and the world over say that exercise is the closest thing to an anti-ageing pill that is available, because muscles can be rejuvenated by exercise, giving them tone and making them stronger. The woman who exercises consistently will be limber and supple. Exercise also counteracts many of the effects of arthritis and keeps arthritic joints more supple.

OUTDOOR EXERCISES

If you do not like doing exercises, outdoor sports can be just as good for you, but do not rely on weekend sport to provide all your exercises—even professional sportsmen need additional exercise to keep fit and improve their game.

Cycling

Cycling is an excellent exercise for firming your legs, from thigh to ankles.

Walking and Joging

Are excellent exercises to tone body and for firming.

Ball Games

Such as tennis, bowling, badminton, basket-ball, or squash are good body stretchers. These sports are wonderful for firming the upper arms and bust, and for trimming the waist line.

Golfing

Has many advantages—it trims your waist line, keeps you out, walking in the fresh air, stretches your body, helps to develop good body coordination, and takes your mind off your problems.

Swimming

Is well known for toning up the pectoral muscles that support the bust: it also firms the upper arms and keeps the body flexible. It is a bit tiring at first but keep it up. (This exercise develops your muscle girdle and helps to reduce your hips).

EVERDAY EXERCISES

As a working wife and mother myself, I know the importance of exercises that are easy as well as effective so that most of the exercise routines can be done while you are watching television, reading a magazine, talking on the phone, playing cards, etc. Begin with five to ten minute sessions and increase the length of your sessions as your body grows accustomed to conditioning.

You don't need special clothing to exercise. Any thing that's comfortable and permits freedom of movement is fine. For on-the-floor routines, stretch out on your rug or carpet.

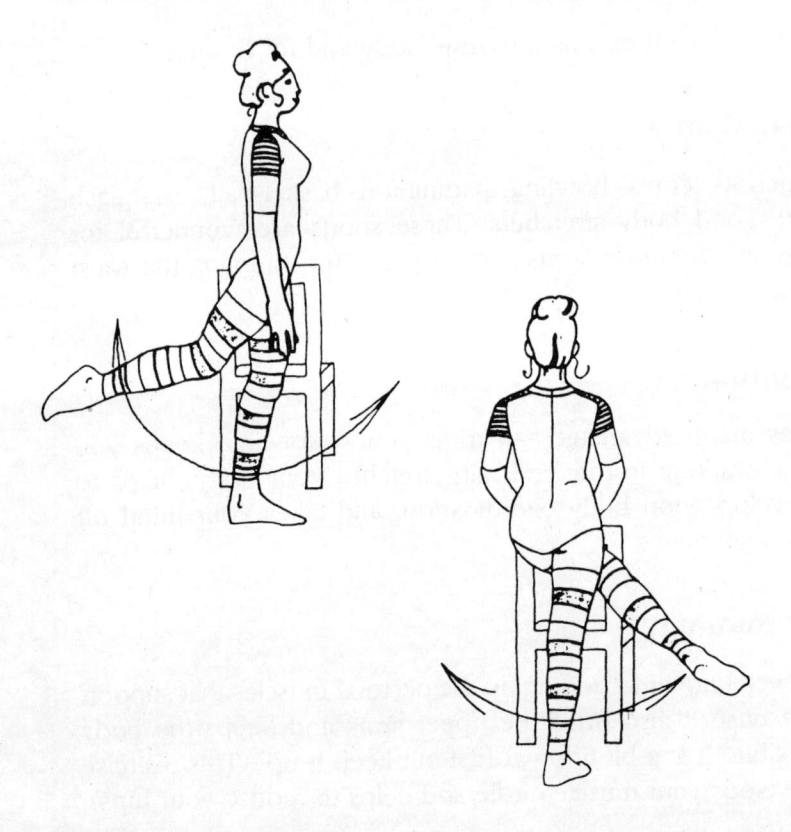

Whenever you do any job that requires bending like opening lower drawers of dressers or file cabinets, dusting furniture legs or making beds, etc., give your thigh muscles a work out by doing a deep knee bend: keeping back straight, bend knees and lower body onto heels, while reaching for the item you want.

Exercise your abdominal muscles while sewing, knitting, reading, watching T.V. Simply lift one leg, straighten it parallel to the floor, raise it as high as you can. Lower. Repeat with your other leg.

Reaching for the highest shelf and putting up curtains also are fine stretching exercise that help tone body and arms. As you reach up, tuck your bottom in and rise on your toes and give a good all over s-t-r-e-t-c-h.

All sweeping movements with a broom are good arm exercises, keeping your upper arm muscles firm and round. Use your arms alternately so that both are exercised equally.

Another exercise to firm flabby upper arms can be done when you wake up and at bedtime. Stretch out on your back in bed with arms straight down at your sides. Spread your fingers and bend them slightly to form claws with the palms facing downwards. Press down with your hands as if you were trying to push your fingers right through the mattress, holding the pressure for a slow count of 3. Relax. Repeat the exercise three times.

You can exercise your waist while on the telephone. Start by bending forward from the hips and bouncing up and down, letting the hand that is not holding the telephone hang down. After a few bounces, straighten up, pull in your stomach, tighten your bottom and then repeat holding the telephone in the other hand. Now bend to the side seeing how far down the leg your hand can reach. Bounce sideways a few times. Repeat bending on the other side.

To help firm buttocks and hips while watching T.V., knitting or reading, sit in a straight-backed hard chair. Sit forward so that your back can be held straight. Now lift your right leg, slowly bending the knee, pointing toes down and lifting the leg as high as possible without straining. Hold for a while, then return leg slowly to original position. Do the same exercise with the left leg. Repeat five times with each leg.

For flabby thighs and bottom, sit on a hard chair at home and at work, and practise tensing up those thigh muscles for a count of six at least 20 times a day. At bath time, pinch fatty areas, after soaping, with a light but firm pressure, giving yourself a massage with talcum powder afterwards.

While waiting for water to boil, exercise calves and thighs by rising on your toes then bending your knees until you are almost in a sitting position (while staying on your toes). Rise again, and keeping still on your toes, bend. Keep on repeating till the water boils.

You can win at bridge or rummy and still work off a dowager's hump at the same time. Pull up from your diaphragm and bring cards level with eyes. This is the correct sitting position. While cards are being dealt, toss head back as far as possible, then drop chin to chest.

Bathe beautifully with stretching motions that help maintain your waistline.

Stand tall to wash your back, then reach far down your back with one arm, then with the other, keep legs straight and reach from the waist to wash ankles and toes. Between latherings, place the soap just out of reach so that you must stretch for it.

Always try to keep your abdomen pulled in as if you were trying to make your stomach touch your spine. This, done constantly, will strengthen your muscles in the area and flatten your stomach.

Appendix I

Diet for Skin

Your skin is a true reflection of your inner health. Anything wrong inside is bound to show outside.

A well-planned menu comprising a sensible and well-balanced diet ranks foremost in the skin-care regime. To realise the impact of the diet on skin, it is important to be informed on what the inadequacies and deficiencies in diet can bring on us.

Deficiency	Consequence
1. Vitamin A	• Thickening of skin of texture • Wrinkles • Aggravation of acne
2. Vitamin B Complex	• Skin pallor • Pigmentation • Dark circles under eyes
3. Vitamin C	• Acne problem • Uneven lightening of skin colour
4. Vitamin E	• Pigmentation
5. Proteins	• Loss of skin rejuvenation. Degeneration of the connective tissue underneath the skin surface

6. Minerals —
   Zinc, Calcium
   and Iron
7. Oil and Moisture

- Skin pallor
- Spot discolouration
- Excessive skin dryness and chapping.

There is no one particular food that can singularly provide all the essential ingredients for your health. A well-balanced diet comprises a host of different kinds foods. Bear in mind that each food item in assortment is rich in one or two of the essential ingredients.

To help you design a menu, both tasteful and healthy, here's a list of various food items and the nutrition value they bear. An assortment of these items can truly make a gourmet meal.

1. *Vitamin A*

Fish liver oil
Butter
Liver

2. *Carotene*

Carrots
Leafy vegetables
Red and yellow sweet potatoes

3. *Vitamin B*

Whole wheat
Pulses
Rice (parboiled, home-pounded)

4. *Vitamin C*

Oranges, Lemon
Leafy vegetables
Guava

5. *Vitamin D*
Fish liver oil
Egg yolk
Butter

6. *Vitamin E*
Sunflower oil
Palm oil
Margarine

7. *Vitamin K*
Cabbage, spinach
Lettuce
Beef liver

8. *Proteins*
Soyabeans, Meat, Fish
Skimmed cow's milk
Beans and Peas

9. *Calcium*
Cheese—Hard and soft
Milk—Cow's (fresh)
Various nuts

10. *Iron*
Liver, Eggs
Pulses
Green leafy vegetables (Raw)

Appendix II

Diet for Hair

A nutritious diet is essential for our growth, well-being and long life. The same is true for the hair. Since hair is the least important of all the human organs, it gets the minimum nutrition from the blood that which is left over after the needs of the vital organs—the heart, lungs and liver. Therefore hair displays the first signs of nutritional deficiency of the body when it occurs.

Hair is an extension of your skin and is composed of cells that have risen from generative cells deeper within the body-cells which are formed, some four to six weeks earlier.

Since hair is made up of protein called *keratin* hair needs protein for its growth and well-being. Now here are some super protein food items apart from meat, that are good for your hair. Scientists have come up with a way of assessing which protein foods are better than others. Their frame of reference is termed "biological value" and the basic is the amount of food required to meet human needs.

Eggs: Have the largest amino acid *methionine* than any other complete protein. In addition, eggs contain large quantities of Vitamins A, B, D and E and many minerals including sulphur. One egg a day can give a real boost to your hair.

Milk: Milk is not just for kids, it's for everyone. It is a complete protein with built-in extra vitamins and minerals that spell lovely hair. All adults should have one glass of milk a day-plus one serving of *paneer* (cottage cheese), ice cream or *Dahi*.

Yoghurt (*Dahi*) is the oldest health food. It contains lactic acid and possesses all the nutrients and proteins in a form which can be easily assimilated by most people. *Dahi* has large amounts of Vitamin B Complex along with bacteria which aids digestion and elimination.

It is suggested that those on antibiotics should have a cup of *Dahi* every day as antibiotics kill the useful bacteria which our hair and skin need.

Sunflower Seeds is low in calories and a good source of complete protein, high in poly-unsaturated fatty acids and rich in vitamins and minerals.

Vitamins: If you are eating well, it should not be necessary to take vitamin or mineral supplements. Vitamins A, D, E and K can cause liver damage if taken in excess. The B group of vitamins, however, are water-soluble and the body will take up only what it requires. Vitamin B is essential for healthy skin and hair and has been considered "food for the nerves" as well as being used to relieve some forms of pre-menstrual tension. So a daily dose of yeast tablets is useful.

Yeast: The composition of a yeast cell is very similar to the composition of the cells that make up the human body. It is a tremendous source of protein and Vitamin B.

Hair Enemies: Actually, the enemies of your hair are also the enemies of your health. When planning your diet, remember that much of what we eat contains toxins and toxic substances. This does not mean that they are poisonous as such, but just that they contain certain ingredients that the body does not need or cannot use. These have to be removed from the body, and the organs through which they are excreted include the liver, kidneys, bowel, lungs and sweat glands. Too many toxins can overwork these organs, causing ill-health, early signs of which could be in the case of the hair and scalp, reduced hair growth, excessive oiliness or dandruff.

A diet high in snack foods, potato chips, cakes, pastries, white bread, foods with high level carbohydrates, sugar-laden soft drinks containing refined sugar or artificial sweeteners or preservative, flavouring and colour, fizzy drinks and fake orange and lemon juice. Factory farmed meats and vegetables can also be high in toxins although these are often difficult to avoid when shopping at the local super-market.